SHIFT

4 STEPS TO PERSONAL EMPOWERMENT

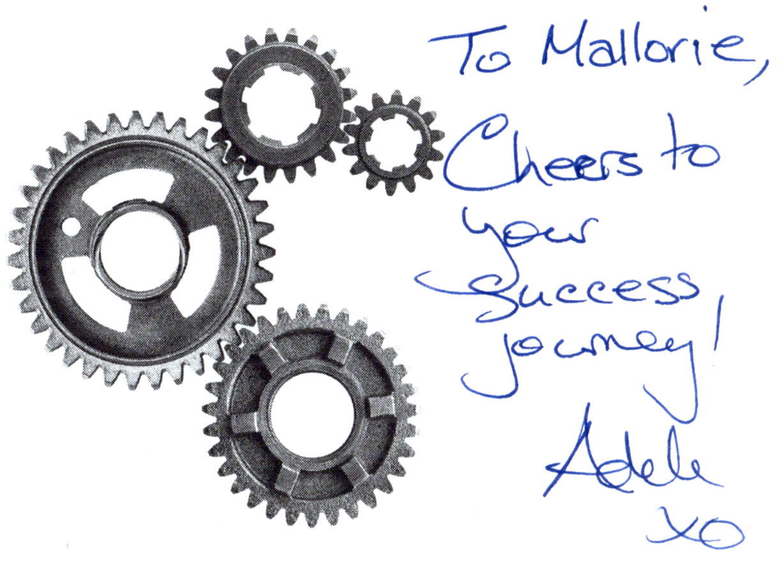

ADELE SPRAGGON

AUTHOR DISCLAIMER

The case histories found within this text are based on real people who utilized the 4-step Repatterning Technique. The relevant facts are real, but in all cases we have changed names to respect the privacy of the individuals.

Printed in Canada

Third Edition, 2019

ISBN 978-0-9919369-2-2

Adele Spraggon Publications

3 Beech Street,

Markham, ON. L3P 2A1

www.AdeleSpraggon.com

To my husband, with love ...

and to all my friends who
will never read this book.

*There is no shame in your past,
no blame in your future, and
nothing to fix in the present.*

*There are only patterns, and
patterns can be changed.*

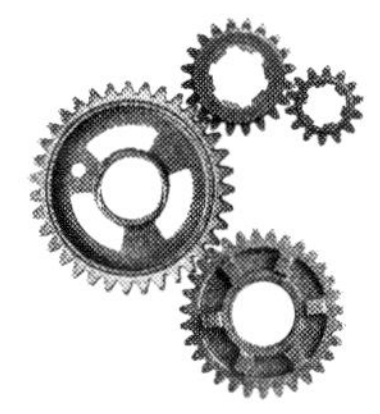

CONTENTS

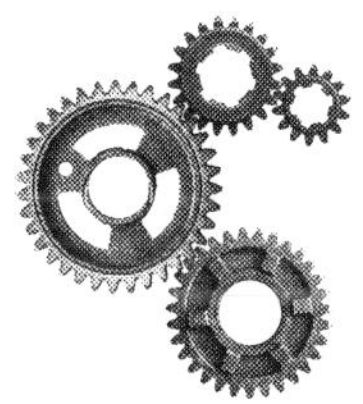

Introduction: And so it begins

What would be possible if you saw the world differently?

What would change if you could stop making the same mistakes, again and again?

What would you be doing if you could stop fearing or doubting yourself?

These were the questions I was asking myself the night I quit my *third* business.

That night I awoke to a familiar feeling of panic starting to wash over me. Panic was something I had come to know all too well over the decades, and it was strongest after I had done something that had me tossing and turning in my sheets, such as I had done that afternoon when I walked away from yet another business partner.

I had two choices, lie there and give in to the panic or get up and move. I chose the latter.

Quitting the first business had seemed like a reasonable thing to do. I recalled feeling compelled to walk away after someone (a stranger at that) had made a negative comment about my initiative. That comment had stung! -- Enough to convince me that the business idea was no good. However, tonight, as I reflected, I could see how crazy my thinking had been as all the evidence pointed to the contrary. The business had been featured on CBC news and had attracted the attention of an international sponsor. Rationality had obviously not been part of my decision-making process.

Ditto for the second time I quit. Again, other people's opinions weighed heavily on my mind. Again, the idea that I was displeasing others had generated a feeling of panic that had caused me to quit.

And now, here I was, having done it for the third time. Three viable ideas. Three different business partners. A number of sponsors. I had turned my back on all of them, leaving chaos, anger and frustration in my wake.

Surely, I thought, it couldn't be solely my fault? I had spent decades exploring, and applying, countless traditional and alternative therapies. Why had none of them been effective?

And so I went to work, with an open mind. I drew on what I had learned as a meditation facilitator and my Masters in Humanities, both of which provided me plenty of opportunities to study the human mind, both subjectively through my meditation, and objectively through my studies and working with my students. In short, I turned myself into an object of study.

The immediate question for me was: why was I quitting and making the same mistake, again and again. So many others I met described the same pattern. They tried hard, and they tried everything: mindset tools and techniques; raising the level of commitment; applying willpower;

setting better goals; being held accountable. None of it worked, and they were no closer to their ultimate goal: happiness and success?

And so it began. A deep dive into my own mind, grounded in more than three decades of meditation. What I found ended my long-life struggle with poor and ineffective patterns -- and now I am helping thousands of people around the world do the same. It doesn't matter where in the world they live or what the issue is that they are facing, the technique outlined in this book helps them to reach their goals.

Briefly, here is what I discovered: At an early stage, in every person's life, they encounter challenges, and they deal with them. Sometimes well, but there is also a good chance that the actions taken to deal with those initial challenges were not good. Some could have been downright destructive like my quitting was for me.

Upon reflection, that person may have thought, 'oh, that didn't work, I won't do that again'. But unfortunately, that's not the way your subconscious works. Because those decisions – all of them – got saved, much like files get saved on a computer. Each decision, the good, the bad, the ugly, formed a pattern in your brain that continues to this day.

Once that decision-making pattern gets stored, it is saved and available for recall. My pattern was responsible for my quitting over and over again. It had nothing to do with the situation, or the other people (my partners or my sponsors, for example), it had nothing to do with my ability to run the business. The reason I was quitting was that I had a ready-made decision-making pattern, stored in my brain and available for recall anytime I had to decide -- quit or don't quit. And we know how that went. Quit.

So all the personal development methods I was taught, all the business tools I was provided, had one thing missing. It was impossible for me to be fully free of the desire to quit, while that pattern of quitting remained in my subconscious programming. Everything I had been taught was missing the fundamental and necessary step of removing what wasn't working first.

It is said that that definition of insanity is taking the same action over and over again expecting different results. This is not the definition of insanity, but it is the definition of past created, ineffective, decision-making patterns.

Given this, I went to work. Again using myself as the subject of study, I created a technique to remove the old decision-making patterns and upgrade them with new ones. It wasn't quick, and it wasn't easy, but it worked!

I call this technique the Four Step Repatterning Technique and one day after I had been using this technique for a few weeks, I noticed something remarkable: the idea of quitting had just disappeared from within me.

I wasn't fighting myself or hanging on in an attempt not to quit. I was not trying to convince myself I wasn't a quitter using techniques such as affirmations and positive thinking. I wasn't looking to others to hold me accountable. I wasn't digging into my past to understand the origins of quitting and analysing why I quit. It was nothing like anything I had experienced prior.

Instead, it was as if I had stepped out of an identity in which quitting was a possibility into another identity in which quitting just wasn't. The idea of quitting just no longer entered my head. It was that effective and that powerful.

That was ten years ago, and I have not quit anything since. Today I have a thriving business that teaches thousands of people around the globe how to transform their lives and the lives of others using Repatterning.

Having now understood the root of the problem, I saw that there are two implications, and I was excited about both. First of all, I saw that there are a predictability and a pattern to the way we as humans react in the situations that come up in our lives – that our reactions are not a result of the people or situations that happen outside of us; instead, they come from the patterns we have stored within. And that means you don't have to blame yourself or beat yourself up if you can't stop repeating a certain behaviour, or thinking a certain thought, or if you get the same sub-optimal results in an area of your life over and over again. It is just a pattern, and that pattern has nothing to do with you.

Second, and even more exciting, I saw that because everything we do, feel, and think is the results from our stored patterns, then *we can do something about them*. I extrapolated this idea pretty quickly: If all of the results in our lives come from our actions, thoughts and behaviours, and all of our actions, thoughts and behaviours come from our stored patterns in the subconscious parts of our brains, then all we have to do is Repattern. Repatterning the brain automatically leads to new results in our lives.

You see, for millennia we have been taught a flawed premise: human beings have free will and therefore, you ought to be able to set the course for your next action. All of our personal and goal setting development approaches are founded on this flawed premise.

All of the latest discoveries coming out of the field of neuroscience are debunking this belief. Take the recent study done by John Dylan Haynes of Max Planck Institute, in which Dr Haynes proves that a modern brain scanner can see the decision you are about to make before you become consciously aware that you are going to make that decision.

Let's break down what this means; we only think we are in control of our actions, but in reality, it is our patterns that are in control. Although, we are taught that the sequence of events leading up to taking action is to THINK -> FEEL -> ACT, in reality, what happens is this.

We FEEL first (information comes in through the senses, and it changes our body's vibration). That change in body vibration activates a pattern, and that pattern takes action (the same action the pattern took in the past), and we ACT second. That action alerts the conscious mind that something is going on, and the mind then generates a thought in support of the action just taken. We THINK last.

Thought does not activate the sequence; it follows. Rather than thought determining the action we are about to take, the mind catches up to the action just taken.

Neuroscience confirms what I saw a decade ago in my meditative inquiry: To take a different action, we need a different pattern. That is what was missing in all my personal development work, and in all the blaming, shaming, "you should be able to do better" methods we are taught to achieve success.

And this is really good news!

Your brain is built to change. It is always rewiring itself. It happens spontaneously and often. How many times have you surprised yourself and accomplished something that felt out of the ordinary?

Now imagine being able to do that all time, whenever you are taking an unwanted action or adopting a behaviour that doesn't serve you. Or whenever you feel nervous, scared, angry, upset, ineffective, unhappy, and so forth. That is the key to happiness, to reduced conflict, to be able to set and achieve new goals and new ways of being.

Humanity stands on the brink of a revolution. Unlike the political and socioeconomic revolutions of the past, this revolution is different. It is a revolution in the understanding of the very thing that brings us our experience of self and world.

It is nothing short of a revolution of the mind.

It won't be long before it is widely accepted that to take a new action, you will need to change your decision-making patterns. In the meantime, if you are reading this book, you are a pioneer - a trailblazer in this new land.

Welcome to a world in which there is no shame in your past, no blame in your future, and nothing to fix in the present.

You see, the problem is not you. It has never been you. Here's the real and only problem: Nobody, until now, has taught you how to remove obsolete, decision making patterns that are not working.

Change your patterns and everything changes.

Thousands have already done it.

I did it.

You can do it.

Adele xo

WHAT TO EXPECT: THE BENEFITS OF REPATTERNING

Between these covers, you will discover my 4-Step Repatterning Technique, a simple yet highly effective transformative practice.

Before you dive into the world of Repatterning, perhaps you might like to know where you are heading on this journey. Here are just a few of the remarkable benefits you will experience from using this technique:

1. A Remarkable Reduction in Worry and Anxiety

Stress and worry are the results of having concerns about an uncertain future. Letting go of patterns eliminates such concerns. During Repatterning, every new pattern you create is created for the situation you are facing at the time, which makes it optimal for the situation. Which means that no matter what life throws at you, you will respond optimally. Accordingly, as you learn to trust the technique more and more, you will naturally experience a remarkable reduction in worry and anxiety.

2. Happiness

As you will discover throughout the book, patterns work by reducing the complexity of your surroundings down to manageable pieces. As a result, at any given moment, what you notice and what you pay attention to is different from what I notice. Patterns are subjective, meaning that you and I can be in the same situation at the same time but be experiencing it differently. It is patterning; therefore, that is responsible for your personal biases and subjective assumptions. The cause of most conflict is differences in opinions. Imagine being free of these subjective assumptions; imagine being able to know that you are creating your reality. The result of this is liberating. You will be happy – really happy! Knowing you create patterns means that you no longer have to "figure it all out," analyse what is going on or question whether you have it right or wrong. Life unfolds with unbounded joy.

3. Expanded Options and Increased Involvement

Patterns are behind the experience of not being good enough. Deconstructing patterns will free you from this self-doubt. Imagine what your life will be like without that little voice questioning you all the time.

I have included case studies throughout the book so that you can get an idea of the results that others have experienced from using this technique. Although their situations will be different from yours, I invite you to look at how each of the people whose stories I share, moved past where they had previously been stopped. That is the power of stopping this voice: You will be able to take on those big projects that you have always dreamed of but felt held back from doing.

4. Risk-Taking -- Without Taking Risks

Before using the 4-Step Repatterning Technique, I couldn't imagine a world in which risk-taking wouldn't feel risky. Before Repatterning, for example, public speaking terrified me. The only way I knew to speak from a stage was to push past my comfort zone and do it. Repatterning changed all of that. I was still deconstructing as I stepped up to the microphone on the day I was to speak (thank goodness for a two-minute technique that can be done anywhere). Then, as I stepped out onto the stage, my nervousness suddenly vanished. The powerful technique took care of everything. That was the last time I was ever afraid of speaking in public – from the moment I deconstructed it, it disappeared, never to return.

Having this tool in your pocket will have you saying, "Bring it on!" because you'll know how not to let anything ever stop you again. Knowing how to deconstruct patterns means that your fears will no longer stop you, and you won't need the courage to push past them bravely. Instead, whenever there is fear, you will be able to let go of the pattern that is causing the fear and step out with confidence.

5. Self-forgiveness and Forgiveness of Others

Consider for a moment the findings of John Dylan Haynes, as mentioned earlier in the introduction, in which Dr Haynes has discovered that action takes place before you are consciously aware that you are taking that action. Now consider that until you learn this 4-Step Repatterning Technique, you had no way of purposefully changing a pattern, and that pattern was in charge of your action. Can you see how no amount of beating yourself up was ever going to work to change that action? New patterns, take new actions – actions that work and so knowing how to repattern, puts us in the driver's seat once again. As a bonus Repatterning brings with it a beautiful feeling of self-forgiveness and, simultaneously, the forgiveness of others as you come to realise that all action is the result of patterns and not of someone's choosing.

6. Expanded Creativity

Human beings are creative by nature. As you learn to create patterns, you will rediscover your playful, creative self. Who knows where your creativity will show up! Are you an artist, a poet, a writer, an entrepreneur, a world traveller, or perhaps a storyteller?

With this technique, I have seen people experience a rapid expansion in creativity and with it the pure joy that flows out of creating for the sake of creating. Whether you choose to act on this creativity will be up to you, but it will be there if you desire to.

7. Self-confidence and Trust in Yourself

Imagine this: Everything that you have ever read, seen, heard or experienced, directly or indirectly, has been stored within you. Now imagine being able to tap into this vast warehouse and draw forth the optimal pattern for every situation you find yourself in from this moment forward.

Self-trust of this magnitude has to be experienced to be understood. It is more than just self-confidence, increased skill or the ability to problem-solve; it is a deep knowing that is truly rare. Most people, when they start letting go of old patterns, report that their friends and family notice a significant change in them – the deep inner peace that comes from trusting the moment is palpable.

8. Enhanced Relationships

In this book, you will find case-studies about people who have used the technique to transform their relationships for the better. You will meet Sharon who went from being estranged from her sister to having deep compassion for her, Rose who established a new dynamic with her team of work colleagues, and Tom who was able to forgive years of abuse at the hands of his brother. Getting results like these with the technique is not rare; it is commonplace.

Most who apply the technique find their relationship issues effortlessly drop away. That is not to say that all relationships reconcile; some people do find that their relationships ought to end. However, with the technique, the ending of most of those relationships is amicable, without the normal resentment and blame that typically accompanies breakups.

Now that you know where you are going on the journey let's dive into the world of patterns.

PART ONE:
Understanding Patterns

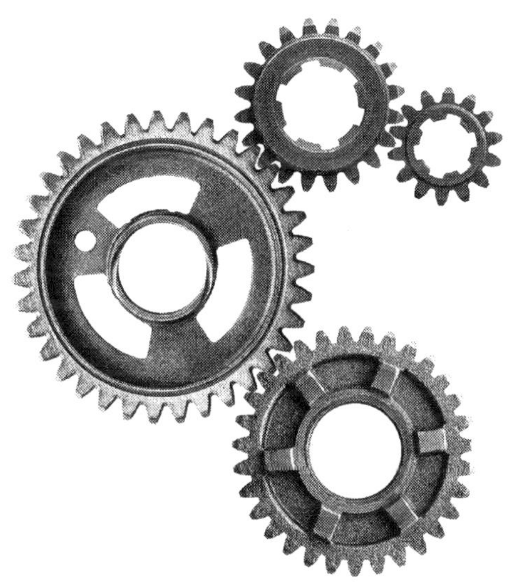

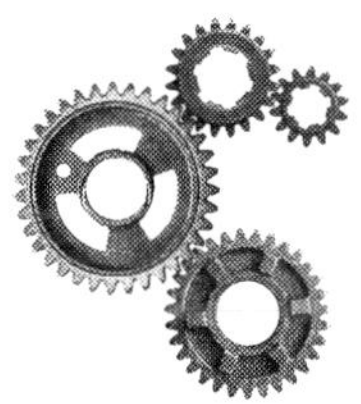

Chapter 1: Patterns, Patterns, Everywhere

Let us begin with an inquiry. What do you see when you look at this picture?

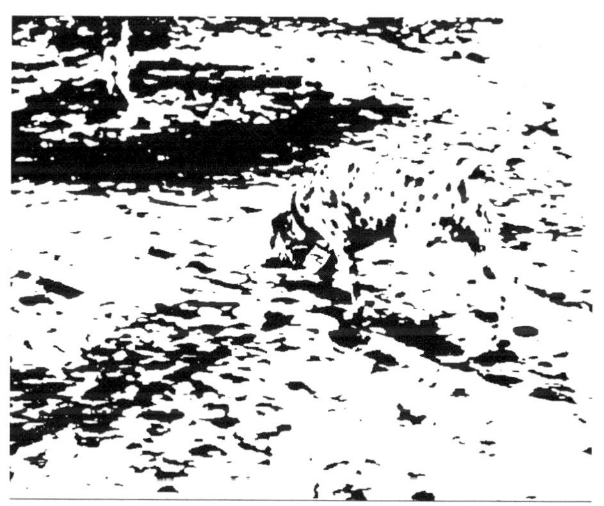

Gregory R. The intelligent eye. New York, McGraw-Hill, 1970

Now, unless you have seen this picture before, it is likely that at first, all you will be able to see is a bunch of dots; but watch as your mind pieces together a pattern.

Take your time. There is a clear and distinct picture among these dots. Do you see it? (If you need a hint, flip to page 6 for the big reveal and then meet me back here).

Congratulations: What you just did was create a pattern. You took what appeared to be random dots, and you turned them into something meaningful.

Human beings do this all the time. We create patterns where none exist: We see elephants and teapots in clouds, men and rabbits live on our moon, and whole villages, birds and mythical creatures dance through the stucco on our ceilings. That is the nature of our brain.

Our brain evolved to take pieces of data and turn them into whole pictures, which is what pattern creation does. This human brain of ours makes associations between events that turn those events into patterns, and it does this so naturally and so quickly that you might miss the enormity of what had to happen for you to be able to see that Dalmatian dog.

Before you could see that dog, you had to take random data (dots on a page) and turn it into something familiar (a dog). You had to take something unknowable and turn it into something knowable – and voila, the meaningless became meaningful.

This natural process is extremely helpful. It means that regardless of how strange and foreign a situation is that you find yourself in, you will find meaning in it, and therefore, will continue to function even in situations of which you have no prior experience. Your patterns provide you with a method through which you can make sense out of the jumble of information that bombards your senses all the time; an ability that is essential to your survival.

However, to really understand patterns, we need to dig a little deeper and ask, how exactly did your brain solve this puzzle? After all, everyone who looks at those dots feels and thinks differently about solving this puzzle, and with good reason, because in efforts to solve this puzzle your brain had to turn to a stored, pre-existing tool available in your subconscious. That tool is your decision-making pattern comprised of a physical sensation, emotion and thought. A pattern that gets activated whenever you encounter a problem-solving situation, such as when you first saw these dots.

What was your pattern for solving this puzzle? Did you tense up? Feel anxious? Think to yourself, *'I am no good at these things'?* Or did you perhaps lean in eagerly, feel a measure of excitement and say to yourself, *I love puzzles?* And then what was the action that followed? Did you go straight to the "big reveal," telling yourself you'll never figure it out? Or did you spend a long time looking at the dots, turning them over and finding all sorts of shapes, refusing to give up until you saw it for yourself? These are all possible patterns that got activated for you when you looked at the dots for the first time.

So let's break this down. My quitting over and over again had nothing to do with my business or the people I was working with; instead, I had a pattern of quitting that my brain kept presenting as the best course of action, regardless of what was going on in real-time in my life. In my case, the decision-making pattern that preceded my decision to quit was 'turning stomach; panic; and 'this sucks, nobody likes it'.

In your case, your reaction to those dots (eagerly leaning in, or anxiously holding back, or whatever else you experienced) was not a result of the dots. Your reaction was instead, the result of a pattern that was created in your past.

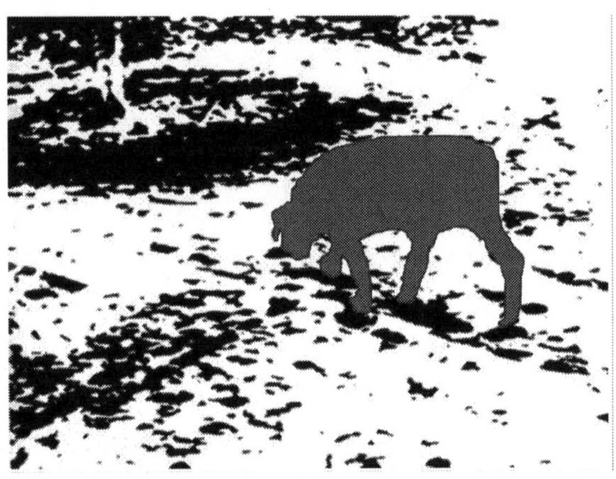

The Big Reveal: The answer to the puzzle found on page 3.

The consequence of this is that you experience the events in your life through a filter given by past-created patterns. Which is why, for example, you might get anxiety when going on a first date with someone, even though you haven't even met them yet – you are simply acting and feeling consistent with an earlier experience. The date you're about to go on, however, might not at all be like the last one, but that doesn't matter to the pattern: The previously created pattern invokes thoughts, emotions and behaviours that are consistent with the experience you had in the past.

Now at this point, you might be considering that patterns are detrimental, and so before we continue, let's explore what the world would be like if your brain couldn't create patterns.

Take a moment to look around the room you are in. Notice how many objects you can see both in front of you and in your peripheral vision. Now drink in as many of the different shapes, colours, movements and shadows as you can. Try not to lose awareness of any one item as you keep adding more and more items and characteristics to your awareness.

If you manage to maintain an awareness of everything you can see, try to include, as well, everything that you hear. For example, you might become aware of the hum of a refrigerator, the roar of traffic in the distance or the whisper of a TV playing softly in another room. Try as best you can to not drop awareness of anything in either field, visionary or auditory. Are you still doing okay?

Increase your level of awareness by adding in touch. Without losing awareness of anything in your field of vision or your field of hearing, add in the touch of the chair under you, your feet touching the floor and your arms resting on your lap.

What do you notice?

Of course, this is an impossible task; most people describe it as feeling like they are about to explode. Human beings have, what is best described, as a "shifting awareness." What this means is that our awareness fades in and out. The more attention we place on one thing, or on one sense, the more other things, and other senses, fade into the background. Not a bad thing; our ability to shift our awareness in this manner is a gift, for, without it, we would be overwhelmed by all of the activity around us and be rendered helpless. This capacity is so central to how we operate and so readily available that we tend to overlook how remarkable it is.

And yet what a keen trick. Did you notice as you drank in the room around you a few moments ago that little of what was occurring was of any relevance to what you were doing? The fact that you tuned out the hum of the refrigerator, the movement of the leaves outside your window and the slight fluctuations in room temperature, allowed you to give your full attention to the task at hand. Truthfully, the majority of what is occurring around you and within you does not require your awareness and therefore it ought to be ignored. It is right that you go about your day mostly unaware of the overwhelming amount of activity (the chaos) that is around you. Creating patterns allows you to get on with things.

Your brain has evolved to create patterns for a reason. If it were not for patterns, action would be impossible. It is not that you would take wrong actions; you would not be able to take any action at all. So, as you can see, pattern creation provides enormous benefits. However, this same phenomenon also inherently has a limitation built into it. Rather than explaining what this limitation is, I'll let you experience it directly for yourself. Now that you have created the Dalmatian, try not to see it:

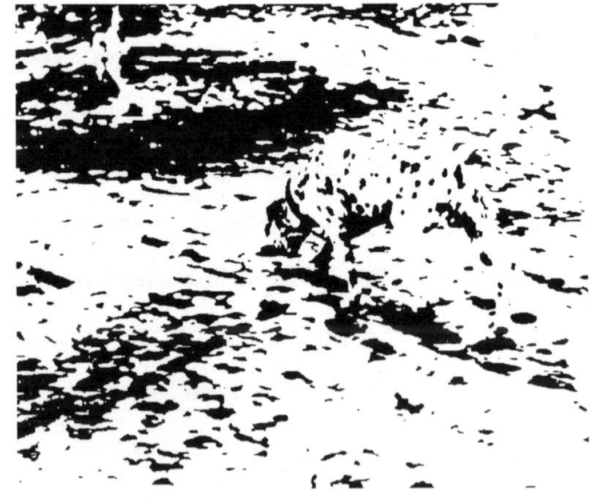

That's not so easy.

You see, creating patterns is the easy part. The difficult part is to *undo* a pattern once you have created it. Having now created your personal Dalmatian, it follows you around, just like any loyal dog. The same effect occurs with all your patterns. Patterns are so persistent in fact, that even if your grown-up, logical self can see that a pattern isn't working, you can't undo it. It's like trying to undo the Dalmatian in the picture once you have seen it.

Let's say you have a fear of public speaking. Fear of public speaking is a pattern. Logically, you may know that standing on a stage can't harm you—that you won't be hurt, killed or maimed—and yet, the fear remains. This is the power of patterns.

Your patterns operate as they do regardless of whether they provide positive or negative outcomes for you. It is of little consequence whether you desire a particular pattern or whether it is working to your benefit or your detriment. Patterns do what patterns do; they run the show.

Patterns explain why people sometimes behave out of character and they help us to understand why two people can be in the same situation and have such different responses. The possibilities within patterns are endless. Patterns are what makes each of us unique: Patterns provide us with our different perspectives. No two of us has the same combination of patterns operating in our subconscious minds. To understand this fully, let's look at how our patterns originate.

THE ORIGIN OF PATTERNS

How and when did you create your pre-existing, decision-making patterns? How did you come to be anxious or confident about problem-solving, convinced you are good or bad at math, eager to do your taxes or able to procrastinate endlessly, or any other of the countless decisions you make every day?

When you were little, your brain automatically created lots of patterns. You didn't have any when you were born, and so each new situation required you to create a brand new response to it. Once you successfully navigated each situation you found yourself in, (and when I say "successfully," I simply mean you survived), you took the pattern that you had formed at that time, and you stored it away for future use. In a remarkably short period (within your childhood years), you assessed the entire world around you, and you created a databank of patterns that you could draw on as you were growing up.

Here is a closer look at how this happens: Pretend for a moment that you are three years old and your father takes you into a large music store. As you enter the store, you find yourself engulfed by the cacophony of sights and sounds. There are instruments everywhere: pianos, guitars, drum sets and string instruments, each strategically placed in their section. Children and adults are coming and going, and raised voices compete within the acoustics.

As you wander the store, distracted by all the commotion, you suddenly find that you are no longer by your father's side. You desperately spin in circles and terror grows in the pit of your stomach. You start to wail.

Decades pass, and you forget all about the minor incident. One day, you enter a kitchen store in search of a new tea kettle and you are impressed by the size of the store. It has kitchen appliances, gadgets, pots and pans and bakeware, all divided by sections. It is close to the holidays, and the store is busier than usual. You periodically hear Christmas carols over the chatter of the many conversations around you.

The store has an interesting layout: Only display items are located at the consumer's level, which means that for you to make a purchase, a store clerk must retrieve the inventory from the upper shelves for you. You wait as the clerk locates the rolling stepladder, positions it in place and climbs the steps to reach for the box you requested high above your head.

As you look up, your mind doesn't consciously register the tattoo of the guitar on the clerk's forearm, revealed as his sleeve pulled back in the stretch, but the pattern running in your subconscious mind picks up on it immediately. Suddenly you feel irritated. You say to yourself that you have places to be. *What a stupid system*, you think. "This is taking far too long." Despite almost having the item in hand, you leave the store without your much-needed kettle.

Let's look at what happened: Walking through the doors your senses drank in the size of the room, the height of the ceiling, the noises, the people, the music, the shadows, the sounds, the smells, and such. Your unconscious mind turned first to your pattern box and selected from that box the pattern that most closely aligned with the situation. In this case, the one your brain selected is the one that was created decades earlier as you had walked through the doors of the music store holding your father's hand.

The slight tension and uneasiness of the pattern went mostly unnoticed; that is until a glimpse of the tattoo in the shape of a guitar reminded the pattern of the guitars in the music store you had walked into so long ago. Suddenly, the pattern reacted, you felt irritated, and you left the shop emptyhanded. None of it was conscious, of course. Your conscious mind didn't even acknowledge the guitar. Patterns occur and operate beneath the surface, in the depths of the psyche too deep to fully understand.

Looking at the two situations side by side, it doesn't make immediate sense how they are connected: You are no longer three years old, a tattoo is not a real guitar, they are two completely different stores, and so on. Even if you *could* remember the incident in the music store (it was forgotten long ago), the connections between the two situations are minor at best.

Regardless, the pattern you created when you were three years old got activated in your mind and caused you to feel irritated, annoyed and anxious. It was the pattern that was running the show, and it was the pattern that caused you to feel like you needed to get out of there as soon as possible; not the store or the situation itself.

As you can see from this example, patterns have their own "logic" which, to your conscious mind, can appear most illogical. For patterns, speed is of the essence: Your brain must reduce the vast amount of data coming at you into something you can understand as fast as you can.

Human beings started creating patterns out of necessity – it was necessary for survival. As we saw earlier, the purpose of creating patterns is for our brains to make sense out of chaos so that we can ascertain what action to take next. It doesn't matter to our brains whether or not the patterns that it runs are "good" or "bad" for us, in the sense of whether or not they are going to help us reach our goals, or whether or not they are going to help us take the most favourable action for ourselves and those around us. In the above example, it didn't matter that you really needed that tea kettle and that it would certainly have been "better" for you to have left the store with it. The pattern acted to remove you from a potentially harmful situation because your subconscious recorded the terror you experienced when you were three years old, and so now there remains a need to protect you from potential harm.

Patterns also don't care whether or not they're accurate. In earlier days of human development, when it came to survival, it wasn't important whether the stripes lurking in the tall grass belonged to a tiger or not; what was important is that you got away fast. If they didn't belong to a tiger, so be it; you got a bit of exercise. If they did, that quick reaction just saved your life. The purpose of patterns is not truth; the purpose of patterns is to turn the unknown into something knowable and to do so in the least amount of time with the least amount of data.

The most efficient way for our brains to do this is to look for and find *what we already know*. For example, if we had to stop to look deeper into that tall grass and ask ourselves, "Hmm.... Is that a tiger or is that grass? Let me take a closer look," we would already be dead. Humans, therefore, mastered responding to the environment using only the smallest bits of data, quickly. Our patterns are not trying to be deceptive; it's simply a matter of survival: react first and figure it out later.

So what's important to note is that there is no moral or value-based compass that your patterns follow. You form patterns for the sake of taking action to keep you safe, and there is a big difference between action and *correct* or *optimal* action.

As you go through this book and learn to work with your patterns, I will remind you of this again and again. There are no inherently "good" patterns or "bad" patterns. Your patterns exist to keep things workable—to support awareness within confusion—and to enable your survival. All patterns are "good" in this sense - they kept you safe at the time they were created, and they continue to ensure your survival today. Keep this in mind as you go through the book. No patterns are wrong; they either work for the given situation you are in, or they don't work up against your goals and what you want for your life.

Now that you are aware of what patterns are, and you know where your patterns came from and how you created them, you can start to assess whether or not the patterns in your current pattern box are useful for you now (workable) or not useful for you anymore (unworkable). Before you can gain the full benefit of being a Pattern Maker, you'll need to know how to recognise the limitations of the patterns you've got stored in your box and so, that is where we will turn to next.

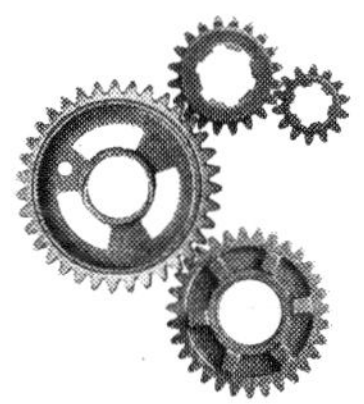

Chapter 2: The Limitations of Past-Created Patterns

On a cold January day at seven-fifteen in the morning in a subway station in Washington D.C., a woman stood, mesmerised, as Joshua Bell's fingers and bow danced over the strings of his Stradivarius, releasing the most exquisite music ever composed for the violin. In total, 1,097 people streamed by, unaware that right in front of them was one of the most famous classical musicians in the world, playing one of the most valuable violins ever produced (his violin alone is estimated to be worth $3.5 million).

A few minutes into the performance, a woman tossed the first dollar bill into his violin case, and two children paused to listen. That was pretty much the extent of the attention he received that day. In the forty-five minutes that Bell played, he collected a total of fifty-nine dollars, mostly in one-dollar increments (excluding the twenty-dollar bill which was given to him by the only woman who had recognised him). Days later, Bell performed at Boston's Symphony Hall to a standing-room-only crowd, where people suppressed their coughs so as not to interrupt the performance; yet that day in the subway station he was just another street performer, barely worth a second glance.

Why?

This example brings to light one of the limitations that patterns carry: In their haste to determine what is necessary for us to be aware of, more often than not, they miss a lot of what is important. Patterns provide us with what can be called *perceived value*. They act as a quick mental shortcut, determining what is worthy of our attention and what is not worthy of our attention. And sadly, all too often, they get it wrong.

Also, recall that all of the patterns in the pattern box got created in the past. Therefore, patterns replace what is going on in the present with what happened in the past. In other words, your world view is not an accurate assessment of what is going on in any given moment; instead, it is a fabrication given by what your past-created patterns *tell you* are going on.

Now, just in case that whizzed by your patterns, I'm going to repeat it because it is super important: *You don't see the world as it is; you see the world as your past-created patterns inform you it is.* Your perception of the situation does not come from what is happening in the actual moment, but instead, from what was going on at the time that pattern got created. This tendency to overriding the present with the past is a nifty trick that we'll explore in detail throughout this book.

The benefit of this is, of course, that fast reaction time; yet this benefit comes at a cost. In the above example, the people walking by Bell as he was performing interpreted his performance through a pattern that they had created in their past. What patterns enabled people to dismiss him that day? Was it the same pattern they relied on to get them to work in the morning? Was it one of "hurried, anxious, I have to catch the train," or, "tired, annoyed, my job sucks?" That pattern served a purpose, but the cost was missing out on seeing one of the best musicians in the world free of charge, and they didn't get to listen to music that could have elevated their moods or changed the trajectory of the rest of their day.

Patterns limit us even when we are not aware they are limiting us. For example, when I first met Brooke, she was not exercising. At one point, I suggested that she take up walking. Brooke's immediate response was, "No, I can't do that. I get winded when I walk."

I knew this to be true. Brooke and I had once walked together from one convention hall to another and inside of just a few minutes, she was huffing and puffing. However, at the same time, I also knew that Brooke ran her own construction company; she was in the business of renovating houses. I asked her, "Do you take sledgehammers to walls?"

"Yes," she admitted.

"And do you get winded?"

"No - but that's different."

"What's different about it?"

"That's work," she responded.

I suggested that 'winded' was a pattern, and sent her off with a homework assignment to go for a walk.

Here is what happened: She put on her running shoes, walked down to the end of her driveway, paused wondering whether to go left or go right and realised she was winded. Laughing, she phoned me and said, "It's a pattern."

Brooke then went on to deconstruct the pattern. The last time I heard from her, she had sent me an email saying that she had just returned from a hiking holiday. She now loves walking.

I love this story because it illustrates quite a bit about the nature of patterns: First, it shows how *real* they can appear. Patterns in the subconscious pattern box are *always* past created - meaning they are never 100% relevant to the situation one is in any given moment.

To the pattern, your thoughts, your feelings, and the actions you take always seem as if they are regarding what is going on around you at the moment. That is what I mean when I say "real." Brooke never considered questioning the fact that she got winded while walking despite her ability to take sledgehammers to walls - and why would she? She got winded walking, and that was a fact. What she couldn't see was that the reason she got winded walking had nothing to do with her body at that moment and everything to do with her *pattern*.

Patterns often—no, *always*—fool you into thinking that their worldview is real. When you feel stressed out, for example, doesn't it appear logical that the source of the stress must be out there, coming from the situation? You are stressed out because of the tight deadline, or your boss who refuses to listen, or the client who is demanding more than you can deliver. What is hidden from you is that the source is never out *there*; the real cause of all of your experiences is always to be found in your patterns.

As Brooke explored her patterns (physical sensations, emotions and thoughts), she gained a valuable insight: Whenever she attempted to do anything for herself, the pattern that got activated triggered the belief or the thought, "I'm selfish." Therefore, whenever Brooke went to exercise—to take care of herself—the pattern caused her to feel "winded."

When I was young, if I was going through a challenge, my grandmother used to say to me, "Adele, the answer is right under your nose, and you can't see it." She was right, and patterns explain why. It is the same reason 1,096 people dismissed Joshua Bell as an average street performer and why Brooke was convinced that walking caused her to get winded.

"Reality," as human beings perceive it, is provided by *our patterns* and not by our situations. The result of this is many of us miss out on life's Stradivarius moments because we're too busy subconsciously reacting to something from our past instead. Did the people rushing to work in the subway that day even hear the music over the clamour of their pattern?

Did you notice the excitement in your six-year-old daughter's eyes as she so proudly held up her finger painting to you? Did you catch the look of disappointment in your spouse's eyes as you brushed off the gift of a single perfect rose? How can we balance these two conflicting needs within us: the need to ignore some things in order to function, and our desire to capture the extraordinary richness of the world around us? To answer this, we will need to delve a little deeper into the world of patterns.

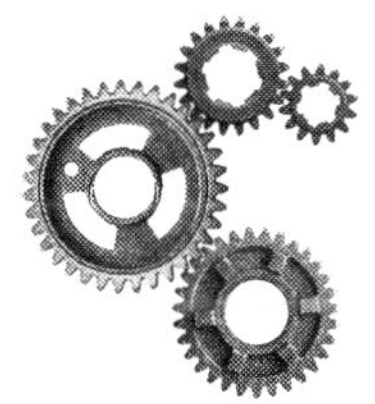

Chapter 3: Optimal, Workable and Unworkable Patterns

A pattern, is a pattern, is a pattern – right? Wait, not so fast. Yes, all patterns consist of a physical sensation, an emotion and a thought, but not every pattern is created equal. There are three types of patterns:

1. **Unworkable: Patterns that are no longer aligned with the situation you are in, and as a result, cause conflict, either internally or externally**
2. **Workable: Patterns that, despite being created in the past for a different situation, continue to be effective in your current situation**
3. **Optimal: Patterns that are aligned perfectly with the situation you are in**

Unworkable patterns will produce destructive results in your life. When I first met her, Georgina was convinced that she was addicted to sugar. She had tried all too many approaches to try to stop eating dessert and candy, to the point that she had all but given up the fight. As a result, she kept candy on her desk, ate dessert after lunch and dinner and, if she had breakfast, it was always a doughnut. Georgina never went a day without eating sugar.

She once said to me, "If you tell me you have a magic wand, and it will stop me from eating dessert, I'm going to ask you not to tap it." For Georgina, life without dessert was just not worth living.

One of the things that stood out for Georgina as she reflected on her relationship to sugar was the way that she behaved in the grocery store. Her favourite part of grocery shopping was always shopping the candy aisle, and she never went into a grocery store without walking down it. At times, she would go to the grocery store for the sole reason of going down that aisle. Because of this unworkable pattern, Georgina felt out of control. She was unhappy with her body, and she was trying to use constraints to fix her problem.

Workable patterns are also past-created, but they just so happen to also fit well with the situation in the present. For example, if you burned your hand on the element of a stove when you were a child, and as an adult, you are careful not to touch the elements on the stove while you're cooking, you could say that that is a workable pattern: It was created in the past, but is still relevant in the present moment. Workable patterns are useful, although they're not optimal, as you'll see below.

Optimal patterns are born out of the situation. Unlike past-created patterns that get activated, optimal patterns are birthed at the moment. As such, they provide the best course of action at the moment, and as you will see a little later in the book, they provide win-win solutions for everyone. They are optimal in that they fit the situation best, and they provide the best possible outcome for all involved.

As Georgina started learning the technique to let go of her patterns, each week, I would gently inquire about how the dessert and candy-eating were going. At first, her response was always the same: No change. But after a few weeks, there came the day that Georgina paused after I asked her the question, and she said with measured surprise in her voice, "You know, come to think of it, I had a bite of pie two days ago, but that's the only dessert I have had all week."

Her surprise grew with the exciting realisation that followed: "Do you know something? The other day, I went to the grocery store, and I walked right past the candy aisle!" As the full realisation hit her, her voice rose with even more excitement: "Adele! I didn't go down the candy aisle!" What struck Georgina is not so much that she hadn't gone down the candy aisle - it was that she hadn't even *noticed* that she hadn't gone down it in the first place. That is an optimal pattern at work!

What makes a pattern optimal? The short answer is that a pattern is optimal only at the time of its creation. For a pattern to be optimal, it must be directly related to the situation you are in the present moment. Optimal patterns are formed *out of* the now and *for* now.

Once an optimal pattern is stored; however, it goes from being optimal to being either workable (it continues to be effective), or unworkable (it results in conflict). (Recall that workable patterns are workable for only one reason: The past continues to align with the present.)

As you start creating optimal patterns, you will likely find that, like Georgina's, they come with an element of surprise. It's not that Georgina was avoiding sugar or trying to control it - she simply didn't think about it anymore. The optimal pattern, birthed out of the situation she was in—shopping in the grocery store—meant that there wasn't a problem to fix.

There is a great deal of difference between creating an optimal pattern and attempting to manage an unworkable pattern. For example, it was clear that quitting was an unworkable pattern for me. It resulted in my leaving perfectly viable businesses simply because that was what my pattern was programmed to do. No amount of trying to manage my tendency to quit was going to "fix" the pattern; patterns cannot be "fixed." My only option was to *dismantle* the unworkable pattern ("quitting") and thereby leave myself room to create something for that situation that was a much better fit for my life and what was important to me. And, as mentioned in the introduction, that was ten years ago, and I have not thought about quitting since that deconstructing that pattern.

How can you tell which kind of pattern you're running? When you are running a workable or optimal pattern, the outcomes are usually positive: they don't result in an internal or external conflict. What you should be interested in, however, is being able to identify when you're running an unworkable pattern, since these are the patterns that you will need to deconstruct. You will know you are running an unworkable; it by one tell-tale sign: "*Something is wrong.*"

"Something is wrong" is a message from your Pattern Maker (the subconscious part of your brain) inviting you to let go of the pattern that is running. It might come in the form of a conflicted emotion or thought such as fear, anxiety, helplessness, shame and the like. It might come in the form of a conflict in your situation, such as when you set a goal and then find yourself procrastinating, or other forms of self-sabotage. It might show up in how you communicate with others, such as going to talk to your teenage son and ending up yelling instead. No matter how you receive the message "something is wrong," it is an indication of only one thing: You are running an unworkable pattern. In other words, the pattern selected from your pattern box is from the past and is out of alignment with the situation you are in at the moment.

As you learn to relate to yourself and your patterns in this way, the message "something is wrong" becomes a welcome one. This message is part of your built-in guidance system, readily available and always present when you need it.

SELF-IMPROVEMENT VS REPATTERNING

Until I understood the different types of patterns and how they work, I, too, tried to manage my unworkable patterns using methods such as goal setting, working on commitment, employing motivational techniques, and so on, all of which would typically provide me with less-than-stellar results. It's not that any of the traditional methods of self-improvement are wrong; it is just that they are not all that effective. Would it surprise you to know that out of the whopping number of people who set New Year's resolutions each year—presumably designed to interrupt unworkable patterns—only 8% achieve their goals? That's eight people out of one hundred! Those are terrible odds. And the sadder fact is I bet you weren't surprised at all.

That's because most people know how ineffective at achieving our goals we humans are, despite the billions of dollars we spend on self-improvement programs annually. The problem with all of the well-meaning advice we hear, and all of the strategies we try to implement, is that they don't take into account the nature of our past-created patterns that run the show again and again, regardless of what our goals are, or how we try to reach them.

Take, for example, a common method you may have learned: *To reach your goals, make a commitment, and stick to it!* Let's explore this together.

THE PERILS OF COMMITMENT

Bishop T.D. Jakes took out a large handkerchief and wiped the sweat from his head and brow in a quick circular motion. What had started as a crisp, white linen suit now clung limply to his bulky frame. He bellowed at his congregation: "It's about commitment! You can have all the education you want, but if you don't commit, you will not succeed!" [1] More than a few heads nodded in agreement.

He continued: "Your life is a false advertisement! Your whole life is a façade—a fake—built on commitments you have never been willing to pay." More heads were by now bobbing up and down, and some of the audience were on their feet, cheering and applauding.

"Commitments have nothing to do with your feelings! Stop expecting to be rewarded for what you are supposed to do." The majority were now on their feet, and loud cheers and laughter rang through the audience. "Say it with me three times: Commitment! Commitment! *COMMITMENT!*"

When I heard Bishop Jakes speaking, I thought of the role commitment has played for me. I have spent a great deal of time and effort trying to follow through on my commitments in my life. Fulfilling on some of these commitments came easily to me. For example, to become a meditation facilitator, I had to attend the temple for three hours every day for a period of six months. To miss more than one day a month was to forfeit the program. I never missed a single day, and my youngest child was two years old at the time. In Kundalini Yoga, the route to mastery is through commitment – a commitment of one-thousand days, to be exact. With gusto, I took on doing a meditation set for one-thousand days. I completed it without a hitch.

However, this ease was not always present in my commitments. For several years, I participated in a popular personal development program that maintained integrity as its foundation. The idea was that once I had given my word, it overrode all else, including my feelings. I thought that I could finally manage my habit of quitting by way of this program, and so I gave my word and faced my fears with ferocity. Did I succeed? Not by a long shot.

To complete the program, I had to pass certain measures. One measure was to enrol someone who had previously attended an introduction into the program. The overall measurement for success was ten percent: For every ten phone calls, I needed one enrollment. Over three months, I made over sixty telephone conversations without a single enrollment.

As the program completion date neared, I voluntarily went to the program centre every single day. When the program ended, I requested an extension, so I could keep trying. Eventually, however, I had no choice but to admit defeat. To pass, I was going to have to acquire a total of nine "yes" responses in a row; a seeming impossibility considering I was zero to eighty.

This experience begs the question: What is missing in Bishop Jakes' philosophy? Why does commitment work in some instances and not in others? And more importantly, should I be placing such a high emphasis on my level of commitment over my feelings? For me, the final result of participating in that program further contributed to my internal conflict. My failure to achieve a single "yes" only fueled my inner critic and further confirmed the already shattered impression I held of myself.

When we attempt to control our patterns through manipulations, we do so at a cost. To navigate around a pattern, we must empower the premise that "something is wrong." Sometimes we decide the thing that is wrong exists *out there* (the boss, the spouse, the world, and so on) and other times, the thing we make wrong is ourselves (I'm not good enough, smart enough, disciplined enough, and so forth.) In my case, as I made call after call, my inner critic did a happy dance at every failed attempt. Rather than dismantle the unworkable pattern of my inner critic rising against me, I tried to silence it, in a feeble attempt to keep going and try to reach my goal.

Looking back, some of the ways I tried to silence my inner critic were quite humorous. Someone once suggested I use visualisation and so I imagined the critic as the wicked witch who held sway over the whole town using her black magic. In a cloud of black smoke, amid loud claps of thunder and lightning, she would mystically appear, sending the town's people scurrying. But then, just as suddenly, the people would turn the tide: They would rise as one and rush at the witch with their torches, scythes and pitchforks, overwhelming her. Following this, she would be escorted to the outskirts of town (usually she was unceremoniously tossed in a wheelbarrow and wheeled out) and left there to perish of her own accord. (Surely, if visualisation worked, this would have done it.)

What methods do you use to attempt to manipulate, or "fix," your patterns? Do you rely on affirmations, visualisations, goal setting, courageously sticking to the task, positive thinking, accountability buddies, gold star rewards, gratitude journals...? As you delve deeper into the world of patterns, it will naturally become clear why some of the things you commit to doing come easily and why sometimes commitment backfires. It has nothing to do with your skills and abilities, and everything to do with the fact that your patterns are unworkable and cannot be "fixed" through manipulations of the conscious mind. When your patterns conflict with your goals or with the situation at hand, there is no way you can succeed using manipulations.

Although he wasn't aware of this, Bishop Jakes' patterns were supporting him all the while. Near the end of his sermon, he revealed the following history:

> *When I started my church, I didn't have anything! We worked when we didn't have food; we worked when we didn't have lights. I only had one suit. I had to wash my suit in the washing machine. They laughed at me! They said I looked like a country preacher! I had holes in my shoes. They laughed at me. I was embarrassed to kneel down in my own church because I didn't want anyone to see those holes. I don't care what you think – if I believe it, I will be it!*
>
> *Somebody yell commitment. ...You'll never bring down someone*

who is committed because somebody who is committed has been down before they ever got up.

I do not doubt that there were times in the early days of starting his church that Bishop Jakes wanted to give up. But then he would hear someone tittering behind his back, and he would bristle, remembering those who called him a "country preacher." At the end of a very long day, he would remove his shoes and look down at those holes, and he would take off his only suit and place it into the washing machine.

All of those actions would trigger a pattern: a pattern that, in his case, was strengthening—not weakening—his resolve. What pattern was it? Was it one of a set jaw; stubborn; *'I'll show you?'* Did he stand a little taller, plant his rebellious feet firmly in the ground and say to himself, "*You'll never bring me down?*" Bishop Jakes was committed, *but it was his patterns that made his commitment possible*. The reason he kept going was that he had several patterns in his pattern box that would not have it any other way. But—and it's a big but—**without patterns such as these, commitment, will-power, goal setting, and the like, are just self-bullying.**

I advise every one of my clients: Do *not* push past your fears in an attempt to meet your commitments. Your patterns won't allow it. They will pull you back into the safety of that box *every time*. And worse, all of the attempts to go against the pattern will simply further reinforce it. You might make progress *inside* the pattern box, but you'll rarely *break free* of the pattern using methods such as those. It is not a matter of willpower. The answer lies not in fighting your patterns, but in *putting the right pattern in the box*.

And the result of putting the optimal pattern in the box?

It's subtler than you'd think - but the changes are powerful and lasting. With traditional methods of self-improvement, there is an understanding that once a problem is resolved, you will be celebrating, standing at the top of the mountain and yelling out to the world what you have accomplished. That is not the case when you replace unworkable patterns with optimal ones. Instead, what tends to happen is this: You simply stop taking the actions that were associated with your old, unworkable patterns, and then one day, someone says to you, "Hey, didn't you used to...?" You then pause for a moment, trying to reflect on what seems like a far, distant memory (even if your new, optimal pattern is just a few hours old), and with surprise, you say, "Oh - yes, I guess I did." It's seamlessly gone, and you don't even realise it at first. The problem goes from looming as large as Mount Everest to you walking right past it without even noticing that you had, just as Georgina did when she walked past the candy aisle.

So I invite you to take a deep, self-forgiving breath and let go of self-manipulation.

To free you of any more self-bullying, let's start by redefining the message "something is wrong." As Pattern Makers, there is never actually anything "wrong." If you get the message that something is wrong, it simply means you are running a pattern that is not a fit for the situation. It doesn't mean that something is wrong with you, your situations, or the people around you.

The angst that we experience when we get the internal message "something is wrong," causes us to look outside of our self to figure out what is wrong with the people or situations in our lives, or we turn on ourselves and beat ourselves up for something.

"Something is wrong" is not meant to be a value judgment. It is only a signal that you're running an unworkable pattern. This gentle approach allows you to let go of all of your misgivings about yourself and the situation. You become able to say, "It's just a pattern," with a sigh of relief, and precisely because it is "just a pattern," you can let it go, which I'll show you how to do as I walk you through the 4 Step technique.

There is no shame in your past, no blame in your future and nothing to fix in your present. It is all just patterns, and when you know this, you can do something about the ones that aren't working. You can ask yourself: *Are the patterns I'm running providing me with the results I want?* If the answer is no, then you can remove the pattern from the box. But always keep in mind that you, the people in your life and your situations are not wrong; you and they are just using unworkable patterns. It's key to remember that patterns are not wrong; they work or do not work.

I'll never forget the day I grasped the full extent of what was available through Repatterning. After months of doing a deep dive into my mind, I distinctly recall the way the hairs on the back of my neck stood up and the mixture of excitement and anticipation that washed over me. I remember thinking to myself: "You've got to be joking. I've been meditating for over 20 years, and all that time I could have had the same benefits—actually, better—if I'd just let go of my patterns!" I was on the verge of understanding the full benefits of this simple method I'm about to share with you. Little did I know at the time that this method would take me further toward inner peace and moment-to-moment awareness in months than meditation had taken me in decades. The beautiful thing also is you can do it too. Those who continue to use this technique experience this same deep sense of inner peace in just a couple of years

Now that you know about the different types of patterns and how they work, let's look at what is consistent across all patterns: the sequence of how they occur.

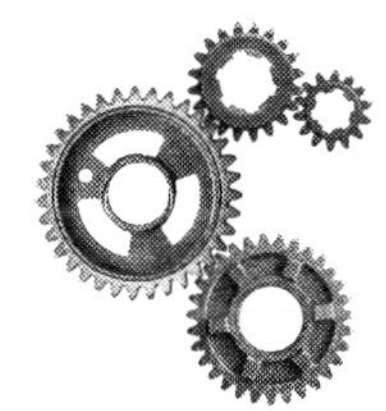

Chapter 4: The Sequence af a Pattern

Recall that a pattern is made up of three components: a physical sensation, an emotion and a thought. Two of these—the physical sensation and the emotion—originate in your body, and the other one, thought, originates in your mind. There are, of course, many ways to distinguish between the mind and the body, but when it comes to a pattern, you really only need to focus on one simple, yet profound, difference: ***Your mind has access to past, present and future, whereas your body only has access to the present moment.***

MIND WISDOM VS BODY WISDOM

Your mind provides you with a rich world of memory and imagination - you remember the past (memory) and then, by way of imagination, project that past into your future.

Now, funnily enough, this moment—what is going on right here and right now as you're reading this—is of little interest to your mind, and that is the way it should be. Your mind is not designed to spend much time in the present. What your mind is designed to do instead is flit to the past, then flit to the future, then flit back to the past, then flit to imaginings, and then to memories...touching down for a brief second on this moment, only to take off on its wanderings again. As far as your mind is concerned, this moment is relatively unimportant. It has a much more important role: to keep your body safe. To do that it must, as best as it can, try to predict the future based on the information it has retained from the past.

There is also another reason that your mind does not have to worry about what is going on in the present; it relies on your body to do that. Unlike your mind, your body is anchored in the present moment, and as such, it is utterly incapable of accessing *anything* but the present moment.

Need proof? Try this little activity: Recall a time when you were in pain – perhaps a recent headache, cramping or a twisted back. Now, try to recreate that pain in your body. Notice how you can remember where you were, who was with you and what you were doing when you had that pain, but try as you might, you will never be able to feel that pain again. It is gone, and once gone, your body cannot hold onto it.

The same is true for any future experience. It is a little subtler, but let's give it a try: Close your eyes and bring your awareness to what is happening in your body. Focusing on any physical sensation you are experiencing at this time will do for this activity. Now, put aside any interference that your mind might be adding, such as thinking about what you're going to eat later for dinner or recalling something someone said to you earlier today. Notice how, as far as your body is concerned, this is it – there is nothing but the sensation you're feeling. Sure, your mind will try to intervene and tell your body that the moment too will change, but by itself, your body can only feel whatever it is feeling. When you stop using your mind and solely experience what is going on in your body, you can see that your body is always here – always in the present. Your body, although mortal, has an experience located in the eternal; it lives in the here and now.

Today, it is a common and pervasive belief that mind prevails over matter. When I say "prevails," I mean that we tend to think that the mind is special in terms of its power and the wisdom it holds. This belief is so pervasive that we no longer even question it, and yet it wasn't always that way. In fact, throughout much of history, our thoughts have not been given much relevance.

THE ORIGINS OF MIND OVER MATTER

As far as we can tell, this now popular belief that the mind's wisdom (the wisdom of retaining knowledge from the past and projecting it out into the future) is superior to body wisdom (the wisdom of the present moment) first came to the fore about 2,500 years ago. A glance through history can help to shed some light on how this happened.

We'll begin in the East with Buddha's teaching that emphasised that "right thought leads to right action." What a novel concept for a time that was steeped in mysticism. *Our future is not dependent on the whims of the Gods? We can plot our own courses of action? Outstanding!*

The West had its glorifiers of right thought as well. Perhaps the best example is René Descartes: "I *think*; therefore, I am." What a pithy little statement. *Thought, and not the musings of the deities, nor our ancestors, nor even our status in society, is responsible for who we are? Glorious!*

And of course, no discussion of mind over body, no matter how brief, would be complete without a nod toward Darwin. *Oh, what shock; what horror. Human beings, descendants of apes? No, that can't be!* If we are no longer to be seen as uniquely created in God's image, there must be some other means for us to stand apart from these homely origins. Mind over matter: that's the ticket — human consciousness. Thought will replace our theories of God. *Viva la difference!*

And so it began: the ever-increasing, upward trajectory of mind over body, augmented in our modern times with theories such as those presented by Napoleon Hill in his popular book, Think and Grow Rich, by books such as *The Secret*, and by philosophies such as the Law of Attraction (the word "Law" always, by the way, depicted with a capital "L" to give it authority). Positive thinking today is the name of the game, right thought not only equalling the right action but also right being, right success, right prosperity, right happiness and even right health.

I suggest it is time we take a close and hard look at the commonly-accepted and pervasive belief that mind is superior over body because it comes with a steep cost to our relationship to ourselves - a cost that becomes more prominent with each passing day.

WHY THE BELIEF THAT MIND IS OVER MATTER NEEDS TO CHANGE

Let's take a moment to look back through time. It wasn't all that long ago—a few generations at most—that if someone were an average person living an average life, they would be able to predict their future by what had happened to them the day before.

With very few exceptions, people's days were consistent: They would wake up at the same time every day, follow a familiar routine, and then retire at the same time they had the day before. The structure of one day resembled every other day. The routine that people followed was the same routine their parents followed, and their parents before that.

Their careers were pre-determined. It was the same job their mothers' and fathers' had, which was the same job their parents' had before them. There were no questions like, "Who are you?" or, "What will you do with your life?" Those questions were best left up to the philosophers. People knew who they were: God and their lineage had ordained it. There was nothing to question and nothing to consider. Life was, shall we say, predictably boring.

Now let's return to the current day and turn in the other direction, outward, toward the future. Notice that everything about the future now exists in uncertainty. The routine, predictable life that people used to rely on to inform them what actions they needed to take, or what beliefs they should embrace, is gone.

"What do we need to know?" we ask nowadays. "What questions should we even be asking? What knowledge do we have today that we will use tomorrow?" And the fact that we can't easily answer these questions makes us realise that the future is no longer lining up so neatly with the past. Today, we might be able to guess what tomorrow will bring, but it will be just that —a guess—because the predictability that the past used to offer is no longer available to us. What will life be like fifty years from now, twenty years from now, or even ten years from now?

As we stand here, in this extraordinary moment called the present, turning one way to look into the past and the other way to look into the future, it dawns on us that this moment in history can be best described as a rupture in time. It is a time in which the past looks and feels one way and the future another.

Now let's turn inward to our boxes of patterns. In this sped-up world, the boxes of patterns that we created in our childhoods and continue to rely on are becoming increasingly obsolete with each passing year. In generations past, people could complete their pattern box in their early years, and then continue to rely on those same patterns as they went through their adult years. That made a great deal of sense; after all, the world was predictable and stable, and even the worldliest of people had enough workable patterns to support them on their travels.

Today is different. Most of us can no longer rely on those boxes we created when we were young to bring us an accurate understanding of what is going on around us.

Every age has its plagues, and ours is no different. Depression, stress and psychological illnesses are at epidemic proportions and rising. Nervous disorders such as fibromyalgia and chronic fatigue syndrome have appeared on the scene. Substance abuses, addictions to internet surfing and video gaming, emotional eating and the like are also on the rise, demonstrating our mind's desire to escape. Mostly, our minds are scared. They are not equipped to deal with this level of change. Reliance solely on our mind's way of operating in this sped-up world is cruel and counterproductive.

And so we stand at an interesting crossroads: If we are going to survive these times with our minds and nervous systems intact, we need to find a new way to navigate through these times of turbulent change. Understanding the true sequence of a pattern can help us do this.

HOW PATTERNS OPERATE

You have likely learned that your thoughts give rise to your emotions. For example, were you taught that the butterflies in your stomach as you approach the microphone are a result of what is going on in your head and that you ought to be able to feel relaxed by generating "happy thoughts."? Let's take a closer look to see what is really going on.

I suffered from panic attacks for decades. Sometimes the attacks would take place during the day, but for the most part, they happened at night. In point of fact, I experienced panic attacks with maddening consistency every night at two am for over ten years. One particular night, however, something different happened.

I was drawn to meditation in my mid-twenties and took to it in earnest once the panic attacks set in after the birth of my daughter. As the familiar panic attack started that night, my then-strengthened meditative mind immediately went into action, and I found myself observing the panic unfolding rather than getting swept up into it. The ability to observe at this level is interesting. I found myself of two minds: While one mind was swept up in the panic, the other observed with neutrality, and in this heightened state of awareness, everything slowed right down.

My meditative mind observed my stomach flipping sickeningly and observed cold beads of sweat breaking out on my forehead. It watched as a rigid tension glued my body to the bed despite my desperate desire to run away. Emotions then followed these physical sensations. My body's rapidly-escalating anxiety moved to fear and then further escalated to terror. Then I watched in surprise as *it was only at this point that my mind was asked to participate*.

The best way to describe what happened is to say my body alerted my mind. Using non-verbal cues, it was communicating the need for the mind's involvement. It was as if it was saying, 'mind, you're needed. *Something is going on*', and then looked to my mind for input to explain the reason that the panic was necessary. If there had been a dialogue between my mind and my body at that moment, I imagine its reply would have been: "Okay body, I see you panicking. I'll check it out – stay tuned."

Following this, my mind did an interesting thing: It began dipping into possibility after possibility, quickly ruling out one before moving on to the next: *Is someone in the house? Are the children safe in bed? Is there a fire?* Once it had ruled out all logical possibilities, my mind moved to the absurd: *Was my husband replaced by a stranger who now lay beside me in bed? Is someone crawling in through the bedroom window? (My bedroom is on the second floor.) Did my youngest child get out of bed, wander outside and drown in the pool? (He was eight at the time.)* Thoughts such as these continued until my mind drew upon the source of my panic. For that night, at least, it was to be my daughter's unusual name and my fear that she would be teased for it.

I have no idea how my mind came to this deduction. There was no logic in its choice. On previous nights, it would have just as easily landed on any other of the possibilities it presented to itself in those early hours of the morning. Logic, it turns out, is not the mind's primary interest.

Wait.... Did you catch that? Your mind doesn't care about logic?! That's right. Although, the reason it doesn't care is most certainly logical: It is not your mind's job to question your body's experience. As far as your mind is concerned, your body's experience is correct. After all, the body is accessing the present moment, what's going on around you. The mind's role, therefore, is to find an *explanation* for your body's experience, not to undermine it. Its job is to *protect* your body, not argue with it. It, therefore, justifies what is happening at the physical and emotional level, but does not seek to change it. And that is why on that particular night, once my mind had determined what it thought the source of the panic was, it relaxed.

Yes, I am aware of the irony: My mind's contribution was to bring my body into a full-blown panic attack by adding fuel to an already escalating fire, and yet it did so with a relaxed awareness that it had done its job. Just before I lost control of my meditative mind and my ability to witness, or observe my panic attack, my mind dropped into what I have come to term "white noise": thoughts tripping over thoughts so quickly that they became indistinguishable. According to my mind, that was as it should be. My body was, after all, panicking. Since my body was experiencing that emotion, there must have been, according to my mind, a reason for that emotion. My mind did what all minds are designed to do: make sense (or if necessary, non-sense) out of what was happening in my body.

As I said earlier in the book, I discovered the sequence of patterns before I could articulate the theory. I now know that *patterns don't originate in the mind; they start in the body*.

I, therefore, illustrate the sequence of a pattern like so:

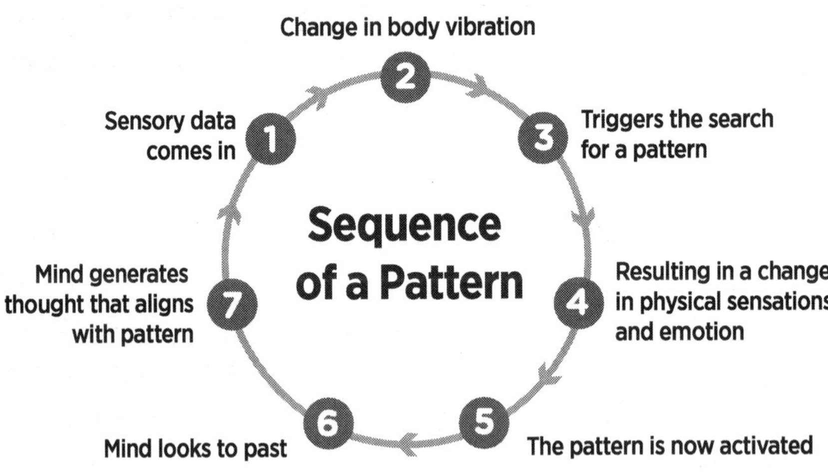

Relating this to your own experience, the first thing that happens in the sequence is you receive an input of sensory data: you see, hear, taste, smell or touch something (#1). That stimulus can be external, such as when you hear a sound, or internal, such as feeling a belly ache.

Regardless of where it originates, the stimulation then affects your body's *vibration* (#2), which results in a change in your body's sensations. Sometimes it is impossible to miss this effect: a loud noise hits your body like a rock, you stumble across something grotesque on the path ahead of you, and a shudder runs through you, or the taste of lemon causes your face to pucker. Other times, this vibrational change can be so subtle that it is imperceptible, and yet, regardless of how aware you are of it, rest assured that your body remains in constant communication with the environment around and within you.

The changes in your body's vibration alerts your unconscious of the possibility for a different pattern (#3 - a "changing of the guard," so to speak), and since the fastest route to action results from an existing pattern, the pattern that is triggered is an existing pattern that aligns most closely with your body's altered vibration.

The triggered pattern, in turn, results in a change in your emotion and physical sensations (#4). If the resulting emotion and physical sensation alter sufficiently, your subconscious will be alerted (#5). If on the other hand, the triggered pattern is not different enough from the one you are using at the time, you will continue doing whatever you are doing, unaware of the multitude of subtle changes occurring in your body.

This multitude of subtle changes that occur between #1 and #4 is happening all the time, resulting in the sequence consistently playing out from #1 to #4 and then returning to #1 again. For example, as you have been reading this book so far, slightly different emotions and physical sensations have been arising and passing and arising and passing in response to your ever-changing environment. However, because these stimuli do not warrant a change in action, you have carried on reading, unaware of the subtle shifts in position that your body has been making or the slight fluctuations in emotion that have been occurring as you have been absorbing this material.

On the other hand, if the triggered pattern does result in a large enough change in emotion and physical sensation (indicating that a different action is required), the first place your subconscious mind turns to in efforts to understand the required action is to the pattern itself (#6). And the resulting thoughts (#7) now align with that pattern, reinforcing the behaviours, beliefs and actions that are familiar to the pattern.

To illustrate how this works: Imagine that you have a deadline in 30 minutes. If you are going to make it, you will need to put aside every distraction for the next half an hour. You commit this to yourself; no emails and no phone messages. You tell yourself just to put your head down and work.

Then the phone rings. You pick it up. "Hello?"

What happened?

Referring to the sequence of the pattern diagram on page 44, the events are such:

1. **The sensory data is the "ring of the telephone."**
2. **Your body immediately responds by sending out neurotransmitters that change its vibration.**

3. **This triggers the search (below your level of awareness) for a pattern that lines up with this vibration.**
4. **You jump a little – your emotion is "urgent".**
5. **The pattern is now activated.**
6. **Your mind looks into the past and FINDS similarities in the present equal to the past; "looks at the phone".**
7. **Your mind generates the thought: I must answer the phone.**

Inside this sequence, it is not until you reached #7—your mind generating a thought—that you become consciously aware that the phone is ringing. Up until then, your subconscious managed all of the affairs of the pattern.

There you have it. It is a simple enough sequence of events; that is until we ask this curious question: *Where in this chain of events did the action of picking up the phone occur?* In other words, at which point did you decide to override your commitment to work without interruption for thirty minutes and pick up the receiver? Did you decide it after #7 – after you had the thought, *I must answer the phone*? That would certainly appear logical, but is it correct?

What I am about to say is now confirmed by neuroscience; however, if I had not witnessed it first-hand in meditation, I would likely approach this theory with my share of scepticism. However, I did witness it, and once I did, I could no longer accept the idea of "mind over matter" so readily. Because as it turns out, *the action comes before awareness*. In other words, you were in action, moving toward that phone, *before you decided to act.*

Inside the sequence of events, action, therefore, takes place here, as indicated in this diagram:

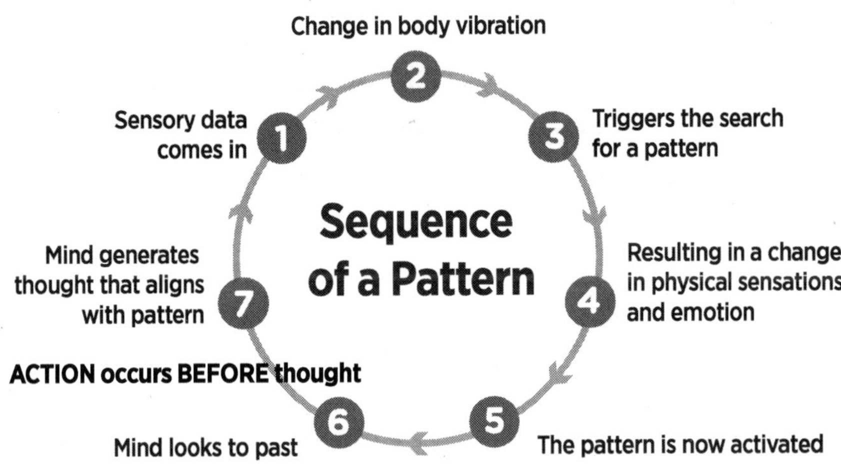

By **action**, I mean an impetus to act: It is a gathering of energy in the direction provided by the pattern. Of course, your hand won't be literally in the cookie jar before you think to yourself, *it would be nice to have a cookie*, but certainly, the *impulse* to take that cookie will be. Your energies are gathered in that direction, causing a change in your beliefs and your behaviours, directing you toward the cookie, causing your mouth to water and your emotion to change to desire.

The definition of action, therefore, can include **your beliefs and your behaviours**, all of which are *previously generated by your patterns and have nothing to do with the thought that follows.*

In other words, *you think in reaction to events that have already occurred*. You think *backwards*. Your mind reflects on the action you have just taken and generates a thought that makes it appear that you had a choice.

Wait! What? The thought is a reflection of what has already happened? The knowledge that you are going to do something comes after you have already started doing it?

Yes, that's right. What the sequence of a pattern shows is this: The thought that caused you to pick up the receiver occurred a fraction of a second *after* you had impulsively moved toward the receiver. Because your mind is not limited to the present moment, it can make a slight jump back through time so that the thought "pick up the receiver" appears to you to be occurring before the action instead of following it.

Now, if you're following closely, you might already have determined why it can be so difficult for human beings to control their actions sometimes. They only believe they have free will, control and the ability to act with autonomy in any given situation. In actuality, they don't.

What happens is that *your pattern* has already decided on your behalf. You behave as if you are the event planner of the party when you are a late arrival to an event that is already well underway.

You are educated to believe that the sequence leading up to you taking an action is: **THINK > FEEL > ACT**

When really, it is: **FEEL > ACT > THINK**

You live in a world that tells you over and over again that you ought to be able to control your actions. You are told repeatedly, that the right thought will provide the right emotion, the right action and, the right result. And so you likely struggle to understand why things don't work out that way: *If everyone else can follow through on their commitments, then why can't I?* And when you cannot, you are left to assume that it must be your fault. The fact of the matter is, the only people who are following through on their commitments, do so, only because they have a pre-existing pattern for commitment.

When you put your conscious self at the pinnacle of your existence, you upset the circular sequence of your patterns and flip it into a perceived hierarchy with your mind positioned as more powerful than, and coming earlier in the sequence than, your body. As a result, instead of your mind supporting your body, it ends up bullying your body into action by delivering a steady diet of "make-wrong" or self-blame.

That, however, is not the design of your conscious mind. Yes, your mind's job is to assess, analyse, label and judge – but when your mind is positioned correctly in the sequence, its functioning is positive, nurturing and supportive. As it is currently positioned, however, it is morphed into the bully.

SELF-BULLYING AND THE MIND

Do you beat yourself up often? Do you say that you are weak and lack self-discipline? Do you tell yourself that you should be doing things a certain way and that you don't understand why you blow it? Given that the answer is in your patterns, it is easy to see why. *Your actions have nothing to do with willpower.* No amount of control would have changed the fact that the phone was already in your hand before you had even thought about picking it up. Your patterns are established at a level below your conscious awareness, and you have no control over the actions that your patterns select. Commitment, willpower, and discipline, therefore, are not the answers.

Which leads to an interesting crossroads: one in which your mind must be repositioned back into its rightful place.

To do this, you must let go of your reliance on your box of past-created patterns. In other words, you must *deconstruct* the patterns that you currently have stored in your box and replace them with optimal patterns that are born out of and directly aligned with your current situation.

We're about to walk through the 4-Step Repatterning Technique together in which you will learn how to deconstruct your patterns.

But first, let's look at what it means to enter the unknown.

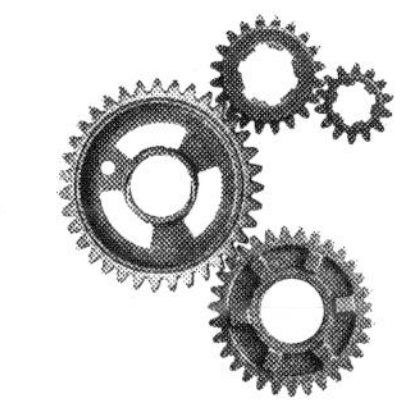

Chapter 5: Entering the Unknown

I could hear the frustration in Mariam's voice as she described her problem to me: "My house is like the Bermuda triangle," she stated emphatically. "Everything that enters here gets lost almost instantly.

"I have multiples of everything," she continued. "I counted: I have twelve calculators. *Twelve!* Do you know why? Because every time I buy one, it just disappears into the chaos and I have to go out and buy another. I've lost things like hands-free phones and even my car keys. This is an extremely expensive problem."

I felt for Mariam. She was a well-educated, top executive in a prestigious firm and yet, despite all of her accolades, keeping a tidy house befuddled her. To make matters worse, Mariam dreamed of having a welcoming home that people would enjoy visiting, and in which she would be proud to entertain.

Like so many of us are taught to do, Mariam had been trying to address the problem as if it lived "out there" in the situation. I asked her what methods she had tried up to that point to address the mess.

"I've hired cleaning persons, but they only clean around the piles of stuff, so that doesn't help. I've bought closet organisers, but they end up breaking under the weight of the stuff I throw on top of them. I have even tried renting a dumpster and throwing everything into the trash - that's how I discovered the twelve calculators, by the way." Even though I knew she was trying to be light about it, there was little humour in her voice.

"Nothing works long term," she continued. "I always end up right back in the place I started." Her voice drooped slightly under the weight of the problem. Now in her early fifties, Mariam was at the point of giving up, worn down by her decades-long attempt to solve the issue.

Why is it so difficult for human beings to take different actions?

What Mariam didn't know is that every suggestion she had heard up to that point in an attempt to fix the problem, whether it had originated within her or was someone else's well-meaning advice, already existed within her pattern box. All the numerous ways that Mariam had tried to address her problem had sounded to her to be viable solutions precisely because she already had an existing pattern that made each solution seem logical.

To understand how this works, we must add to our definition of a pattern. We have already determined a pattern to be an intertwined physical sensation, emotion and thought. Let us now add to this definition by defining a pattern to be an intertwined physical sensation, emotion and thought *that causes the world to appear familiar*.

Recall when you looked around the room at the beginning of reading this book, and you drank in as much as you could through your senses. Do you remember that it didn't take you very long to determine that the task was impossible? Your brain couldn't hold all of that information at once. Instead, it did what all of our brains are designed to do: It shifted awareness. However, what you wouldn't have been able to notice is that what your awareness shifted to was *only those items that had a pre-association with your existing patterns*.

Pretend for a moment that you and I are standing in the same room doing this activity for a second time. Do you think we are both having the same experience? The fact of the matter is, we are not. Later, as we compare notes, you will mention the plant in the corner that needs water, while I will have no recollection of ever having seen it. I, on the other hand, will be able to describe the painting above the piano, whereas you will not recall it. Your patterns will have picked up on certain sounds, smells and sights that my patterns will have overlooked entirely. Similarly, my patterns will have honed in on other items that yours will have overlooked as unimportant.

And what about our impressions of the space? Did we, for example, have the same beliefs about the room? Did we both behave the same way in the room? What did we say to ourselves? You see, everything about the room was not driven by what was *going on in the environment*, but instead driven by *what our patterns determined our experience to be*. What we notice and react to is all given by the patterns that we have in our boxes. If it is familiar to our patterns, it sticks; if it isn't, it goes in one ear, one eye, one nostril, and out the other.

Let's go back to Mariam's story to demonstrate this phenomenon: The only time a suggestion would have sounded viable to Mariam is when the solution already existed inside her box of patterns.

If you have been stuck on anything in your life for any length of time, then you can bet your bottom dollar that the solution is not in your pattern box. However, until you come to understand this, you will keep digging into the same box, hoping to come up with the right answer, and instead, keep pulling out the same old pattern (and with it, its solution) over and over again.

Any solution Mariam tried on—any solution that sounded viable to her—only sounded that way because it supported her existing patterns, and as she attempted each of these solutions and failed, it further verified her belief of being a messy person.

So here we have a catch twenty-two. The only solutions that seem viable to you are ones that already exist in your box of patterns -- and the ones that are in the box don't work.

Knowing this meant one thing and one thing only. Before Mariam could get to the real solution, the first thing she had to do was adopt a strategy of subtraction.

A STRATEGY OF SUBTRACTION

A *strategy of subtraction* is different from the traditional ways of determining solutions. Traditional models are what I call, s*trategies of addition*: In efforts to find the answer to a problem, we keep adding to the complexity of the problem.

In Mariam's case, she added to the complexity by trying to determine such things as; why she was messy, whether or not something happened in her childhood to turn her off cleaning, what the best way to organise the mess was, and so on. She did this by researching, learning, hiring experts, visioning, goal setting, and such. (If these sound familiar, they should. They are all the traditional approaches that we have been taught to use to achieve our goals).

In efforts to distinguish between a strategy of subtraction and a strategy of addition, it is helpful to use the analogy of an iceberg. At the top of the iceberg—the part that is visible above the water—are all of our actions, behaviours and beliefs. Under the water, below the surface, are our patterns: intertwined physical sensations, emotions and thoughts.

We tend to think about patterns in terms of habits, or more broadly, in terms of repetitive things we do, feel or believe. It is important to keep in mind *that these are the results of patterns and not the patterns themselves*.

Patterns exist in the depths of the dark waters, and there they labour away hour after hour. They don't require your conscious awareness; ha - they don't even *want* your conscious awareness. They are much happier if you shine the light of awareness in any direction but theirs.

Now, please don't think of these underwater dwellers as evil - they're the exact opposite: They are fully devoted to your safety. The reason they labour away so diligently is they aim to protect you. They protect your ideals and values, your current status and most importantly, the actions, behaviours and beliefs that derive from your past and therefore appear to you to be the correct course of action. In other words, to protect you, your patterns are keeping you stuck where you are at in the present moment.

Meanwhile, above the surface, all you can see are the ineffective actions (or inactions) you are taking. What you are aware of is the floating ice above the surface: that latest commitment you failed to follow through on, the way you procrastinate, the nervousness you experience on a date, and so on. What is missing from your awareness is what is going on under the water.

As you scramble around at the surface trying to get to a solution to your problems, you do so by reaching outside of yourself for answers. You might enrol in programs, workshop or seminars, or seek knowledge and information by some other means. You might research the internet, read a book, watch an educational video, hire a coach, and so on. Or worse, you might accept that your problem is a limitation in you and look to others to do what you feel you are not capable of doing until you give up altogether.

When you are stuck, all of this frenzy of activity is equivalent to rearranging deck chairs on the Titanic.

The underwater dwellers are still there; the patterns that give rise to your action (or inaction) still exist within you. Therefore, no matter how much you know or learn or wish things to be different, you still will not be able to take the necessary action that will get you to your desired goal.

Now let's compare this approach to a strategy of subtraction.

A strategy of subtraction is different. It begins with the recognition that *you do not have the solution, and it is not forthcoming*. It begins with emptying your cup. You must start from the belief: *I don't know*.

A strategy of subtraction requires that you get to the space of the unknown. The only way to do that is to remove the pattern that is giving rise to the problem in the first place — this approach yields very different results from a strategy of addition. Things suddenly start to change without you even noticing it.

In Mariam's case, after she applied the 4-Step Repatterning Technique for a few weeks, I received a phone call from her. Her voice expressed her puzzlement: "I don't get it. I'm not doing anything, and my house is clean." I laughed because she was cleaning it, of course; it just came so effortlessly to her that she didn't notice she was doing it.

A strategy of subtraction also yields long-term results. Three years after we first worked together, I was in communication with Mariam about something different. In passing, I asked her what she was doing.

"Cleaning," she said.

"Oh," I replied casually. "How's it going?"

"Great! I enjoy cleaning."

I never cease to be amazed at how once an old pattern is gone, it is gone. As the conversation continued, it became clear to me that the anxiety Mariam used to feel about cleaning was a distant memory for her, at best.

THEORY VERSUS TECHNIQUE

In *Part Two* of this book, I have outlined all four steps in the 4-Step Repatterning Technique. I have also provided the corresponding part of the theory under each step. To complete the steps effectively, you will need at least a basic understanding of the theory behind the technique because the mind will not blindly follow something that does not make sense to it. That said, if you are not a fan of theory, feel free to take in only what works for you as you read it.

Think of theory and practice as being in a dance together. If you were to learn something new *without* theory, you would be doing each step by rote (mechanical repetition) and any affects you might otherwise get from the technique would be severely restricted. To get the greatest benefits in *Part Two*, you must know what each step is doing and the impact it is having on your subconscious patterning. Therefore, I recommend that you grapple with the "why" that underlies each step: Play with it, chew it over and ponder it.

That said, the 4 Step Repatterning Technique is something that you will need to experience before you can *fully* understand it. It is more like learning how to swim than learning math: You cannot learn how to swim sitting on the edge of the pool; you have to dive in and get wet. It will take you approximately six-weeks to master this technique.

In going through the different steps to the technique, be patient with yourself. Do you remember what was like learning how to swim? You didn't do it perfectly the first time; you had to learn how to stay afloat, and then how to do the strokes until finally, you were swimming. The steps in this book are the same. At first, going through the technique will feel awkward. You might feel you don't understand it fully or that you're not getting it. All you need to do is keep going. Keep emptying your cup - keep doing the work as designed. The technique does work! Everyone who jumps into the pool gets results. But no amount of intellectual learning alone will give you access to the results.

PART TWO:
The Four-Step Repatterning Technique

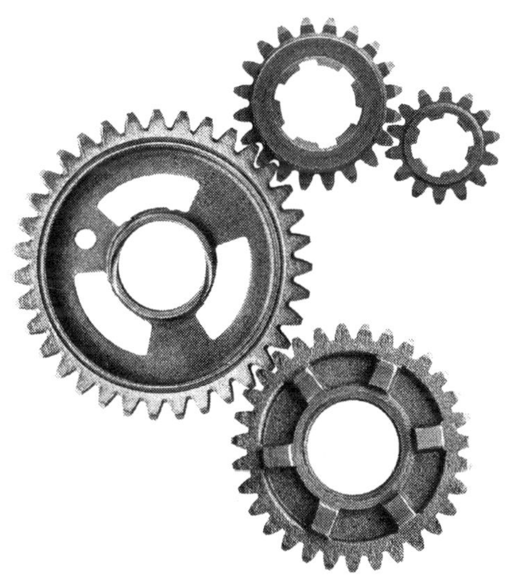

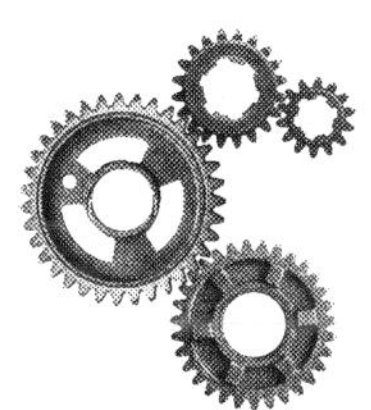

Chapter 6: Step One - Identify The Pattern

Recall that a pattern is an intertwined physical sensation, emotion and thought. In *Step One* of the technique, you identify each part of a pattern. Here's how to do it:

- Start by bringing to mind one of your unworkable beliefs, behaviours or actions. You might have a belief such as, "I need more education before I can apply for that job." You might have a behaviour such as emotional eating, or an action such as harsh words you recently spoke to your spouse. Choose only one of the things.
- Now, holding this in your mind, turn your awareness to your body. Start by identifying the physical sensation that occurs. Where does your awareness go? Perhaps you notice that your stomach is churning or that heat is rising in your body. Maybe you feel slumped or are experiencing a cringing feeling. Don't look for anything special; just become aware of your body's physical sensation as it is occurring. Once you have something, label it; for example, hot, cold, warm, tingling, contracted, clenched, dull, empty, heavy, knotted, numb, bubbly, dizzy, fluttery, pounding, queasy, shaking, butterflies,

churning, electric, sweaty, achy, tender, tense, tight, open, relaxed, floaty, and so on. You are only looking for the main sensation or a maximum of two. If you are experiencing a lot of sensations, label the one or two that are most prominent.

- Having labelled your physical sensation, turn your attention to your emotion. Again, do not look for any particular emotion or what you think that emotion ought to be; instead, only make a note of what is there. Once identified, provide it with a label, such as: sad, happy, angry, disgusted, frustrated, envious, anxious, scared, ornery, proud, excited, confused, panicked, shocked, lonely, rejected, worried, for example.
- Lastly, look to the thought. Make a note of whatever your mind says, such as: "You're no good," or, "what a jerk." Again, make no judgments; focus on awareness. If your mind has no response, you are welcome to use the belief, behaviour or action itself in place of the thought.

As you identify your pattern, consider it only from this present moment. What you don't want to do is try to recall what you were feeling yesterday when you were presenting from the stage, for example. The pattern is running *now*, and so *the only place you can identify from is now*. Therefore, check-in with how your body is responding at *this* moment, as it relates to you recalling being on the stage yesterday. What emotion, physical sensation and thought is occurring *now*?

Here's an example of *Step One* in action: You have just come into a small inheritance, and you and your spouse are trying to decide what to do about it. As far as you are concerned, it is best to put the money into the retirement fund, whereas your spouse wants to go on a vacation. You can feel an argument building, and so you extract yourself from the situation to go and identify the pattern. You are aware of a tension in your shoulders and a tightness in your jaw. After labelling these as: "tension and tightness," you turn your awareness to the emotion. You notice anger, but there is something else there as well – a slight feeling of shame. Although, as far as you know, there is no logical reason to feel shame, you nevertheless label the emotions: "anger and shame." After doing this, make a note of your thought. The thought is: *It's never enough for him*, and you jot that down.

That completes *Step One*.

WHAT STEP ONE DOES

How many times have you been told, "You shouldn't feel that way"? Or, the opposite, how many times have you been allowed to openly express your experience without the person who is listening, attempting to fix you or change that experience?

We grew up in a culture where listening is extremely rare, and very few of us have a role model to follow when it comes to how to do it.

Listening is an opening. It is a space that is created by another for the sole purpose of allowing. That space holds no agenda and no judgment. To listen is to be present; it is generous, kind and loving. And that is the gift you give yourself in *Step One*.

But listening is not a one-way street. To listen is also to acknowledge that you have heard the other person, which is done best by articulating back the emotion that you are hearing expressed. A person trained in listening is taught to respond with a direct and gentle statement that starts with the word "you," such as, "You sound angry," or, "You sound scared." And that is what you do for yourself when you give your feelings a label.

I recall one very poignant telephone call when I was a volunteer on the distress hotlines. The man who called in was frantic. He had returned home to find his wife and his friend in bed together. They had quickly dressed and left, leaving him alone in the house.

His reaction to the situation was scaring him more than the situation itself. In a voice marked by confusion, he exclaimed, "Why am I not angry? Why do I feel this weird elation -- almost euphoria?" His voice was rising dramatically as he said, "What's wrong with me? There's something wrong with me!"

My response was gentle, "You sound shocked," was all I said. With those words, it was as if I had pricked a balloon. A slow, audible exhale, brought the pitch in his voice back to normal, and with noticeable relief, he uttered the words, "Yeah. That's it." When you listen to yourself and acknowledge your experience, you give yourself this same gift.

Labelling provides a connection between your body and your mind. To name something is to demonstrate that you understand it. As you go through *Step One* each time you use the technique, take the time to listen to your body and provide the optimal label for its experience. It's okay to take a stab at it if you are not quite sure what the emotion is.

Listening is not one-sided; both parties contribute to understanding. Therefore, it's a process. Let's say, for example, that I had misinterpreted the man on the phone and instead of saying "shocked," I had said, "excited." He would then have corrected me: "No, that's not it. It's more like ______," and he would have continued to provide clues for us to go on.

So long as you are providing a safe space for exploration, this communication between mind and body happens naturally. Of course, your body cannot respond to you with language, but it does respond. As you get practised in this technique, you'll notice that an accurate label results in a subtle softening in your body. At first, this softening might be so subtle that you don't notice it, yet to your body, the softening is much like the man's audible response of, "Yeah - that's it." It is a recognition that it has been acknowledged and understood.

In addition to all of this, labelling accomplishes one more important task: It anchors your mind in the present moment and what is going on now rather than what happened in the past, or what might happen next. Recall I mentioned earlier that your mind is designed to flit around from past to future. Labelling pauses this tendency and gives your mind an effective way to stay present (typically, body wisdom) that differs from its usual analysis of the situation (mind wisdom).

Having said all that, *Step One* alone will not deconstruct the pattern. The three steps that follow are each vital in the process of letting go of a pattern.

PITFALLS AND HOW TO AVOID THEM

It is not uncommon to overcomplicate this first step. In a culture that is afraid of negative emotions, physical sensations and thoughts, that has confused emotion with action, and that gets uncomfortable in the face of so-called "negative emotions," you have likely been trained to turn away, rather than toward, what is happening inside of you. Therefore, all that you experience is either denied or dulled. Contrary to popular belief, this does not make your feelings go away but has them get buried in the dark waters below the iceberg.

As you begin the journey *into* your patterns and connect to what you are feeling and thinking (not what you expect you *ought* to be thinking and feeling), you allow, sometimes for the very first time, a real-time connection between your body and your mind. For some people, this step can be surprisingly revealing. Your first surprise may be how difficult it is for you to do this first step. Connecting to your body—being aware of its sensations in the present moment—can be a lot harder than it sounds.

It has been my experience that men often struggle with connecting to their bodies in this way more than women do. I can only assume that this is because boys were conditioned from a very early age to deny their body's experience: "Suck it up," "Don't be a pussy *[sic]*," and, "You're a cry-baby," are taunts that almost every man has experienced on a playground, in the sports arena and even at home.

This education away from the experiences of the body in favour of what is going on in your mind takes patience and perseverance to undo. Please be gentle with yourself. If you have trouble locating a feeling or sensation when you do this step, it is not that you can't feel; it all comes back with time and practice.

The other surprise you might encounter when you attempt to label the parts of your patterns is the lack of predictability inside patterns. I'll use an example to illustrate this. Let's say that there is a colleague at work who you find particularly annoying. You might think that every time she enters your office, your pattern will be consistent and that the emotion you will experience is one of annoyance. Then when you start identifying the pattern you are taken aback by its inconsistency: Sometimes you are annoyed, sometimes you feel neutral, and sometimes you feel pity, and then there was that time last week when you felt embarrassed. And that's just the emotional piece of the pattern!

What is going on? Your patterns are only sometimes consistent, but rarely does your conscious mind acknowledge this fact. Even if you are nodding your head in agreement, saying, "Yes, of course. That makes perfect sense. I feel different all the time," your analytical mind will keep imposing its view of consistency over what is going on time and time again. Exploring the moment just as it is, allows your conscious mind to catch up with what your unconscious has been aware of all along, that the present moment is always changing and you, like it, are never the same way twice.

I recommend you spend one week on this first step before adding Step Two. Do this even if you feel you are good at identifying your patterns. The conscious mind needs this amount of time to experience the subconscious, and it needs this week to get used to turning inwards to experience, instead of outwards to explore possible solutions.

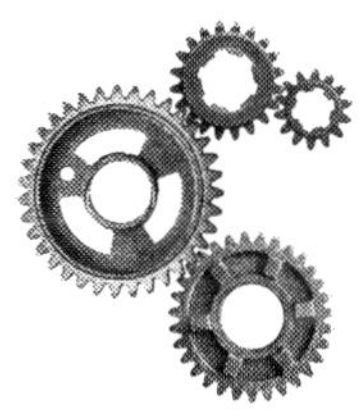

Chapter 7: Step Two - Own the Pattern

Having identified the pattern, you can now move on to Step Two. In this step, you own—or take responsibility for once creating—the pattern. Recall from Part One of this book that patterns all start as optimal patterns because you created them at some point in your past as a response to a situation. To own your patterns is to acknowledge this fact. Here's how to do it:

After you have completed Step One and identified all three parts of the pattern, next, either silently, or out loud, recite the following:

- "**I created the physical sensation**, _______," and then insert the physical sensation that you identified in Step One. Then pause for a second and experience this physical sensation in the body.
- "**I created the emotion**, ________." Name it, pause and find that emotion in the body.
- "**I created the thought**, ________." State it and then notice where that thought lands in the body – there will be a physical response somewhere that results from the thought.
- Lastly, state: "**And because I created the pattern, I can let it go.**"

That completes *Step Two*.

WHAT STEP TWO DOES

How many emotions would you say that you have in a day? How many physical sensations? How many thoughts? The fact is, you have a lot more than you are aware of, and much of what happens in your body happens below your conscious awareness. Your body feels pressure, and it adjusts itself, for example, yet you remain unaware of this adjustment. Your body experiences a moment of sadness, but it passes before your mind can acknowledge "sad." At any given moment, as you go about your day and your night, sensations arise and pass. None of this is the pattern.

The pattern exists in the *intertwining* of your body and your mind. It is the way you *connect* the churning in your stomach, to the emotion "nervousness," and to your experience of being on stage, for example. In reality, there is no relationship between the three parts of the pattern - they are distinct. You don't *have* to be nervous on stage; your stomach need not be flipping, and your thoughts can be directed at the audience and not at your experience. But the pattern doesn't see the world in that light.

As you apply *Step Two*, you learn to own your patterns as patterns and not as reality. As you do so, you put the three parts of your patterns back into their separate components. As you say the first line, you pause to experience the physical sensation for what it is - a physical sensation — ditto for the second line as you pause to experience the emotion as an emotion, and then again, as you pause to experience the thought as a thought. Each piece acknowledged for what it is: an independent phenomenon, separate and distinct from the other two.

Step Two also works at a subconscious level to provide you with a different perspective of your patterns. Recall that the primary purpose of patterns is to reduce the vastness of your situation down into something manageable for your brain. That means that you never have the complete picture of a situation; at any given moment, you only have a partial one. That is difficult for your mind to see. Sure, logically you can argue that you don't know everything, but consider when you are in a disagreement with your neighbour: Isn't your perspective the right perspective and your neighbour the one who doesn't have all the facts?

To own your patterns is to acknowledge the partiality through which you experience the world. This step enables you to acknowledge a pattern as a pattern and not as an objective, outward reality.

Rather than seeing this as a limitation, consider that this is extremely freeing. For decades, Seth struggled to control uninvited thoughts. He was labelled OCD (Obsessive Compulsive Disorder) by his psychiatrist. He tried everything from hypnosis to mindful-based meditation to breathing techniques, none of which worked, and some of which further traumatised him by making him feel that the thoughts, and his inability to fix them, were his faults. The turning point came when he was able to own a pattern as a pattern.

On one of our calls, Seth was explaining how he had spent a few days in nature. Being in nature had previously proven to be especially challenging for Seth, and so I didn't know what to expect next. He was relaxed as he described his experience of his time away. "It's just a pattern," he said casually.

It's just a pattern!

No matter what your experience, *it is always just a pattern*, and because it is a pattern, you can let it go. What you let go of in *Step Two* is your attachment to your patterns as reality and with that attachment, the need to do something to fix it.

PITFALLS AND HOW TO AVOID THEM

The biggest pitfall in *Step Two* can be found in the last sentence of the step when you recite the line, "And because I created it, I can let it go."

The pitfall here is in thinking that you have to *do something* to let it go, or that you have to *know how to let it go.*

It is not your job to let it go! Not only is it not your job to let it go, you actually *cannot.*

"Huh? Wait a minute Adele – you just told me to let it go, and now you're saying I can't let it go".

Yes – that's right.

Because action comes before thought, your conscious mind, by itself, cannot let go of a pattern. I will get deeper into this in future chapters, but for now, know that this statement is a preview of what will come next in *Step Three*. In *Step Three*, I will take you through a special way of observing the pattern so that you relax your mind's need for control. For now, saying "I can let it go" eases your conscious mind by making it think it is in control and giving it its due.

However, don't confuse letting go of a pattern with letting go of your behaviours, actions and beliefs. You are not responsible for the action, behaviour or belief/thought, because *those belong to the pattern*. You are only responsible for the existence of the pattern itself and by "responsible," I mean, you are "able to respond" - i.e. you can do something about it.

As with Step One, it is recommended that you spend a full week applying Step Two to Step One before moving onto Step Three. This time of identifying and owning your patterns is essential if you are going to succeed using this technique. Please don't underestimate the enormity of what you are asking your conscious mind to do, and in the process rush this technique.

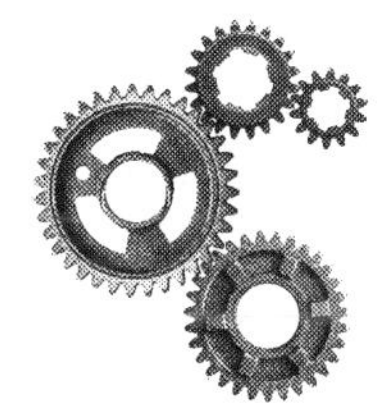

Chapter 8: Step Three - Surrender

Having completed *Step One* in which you identified the pattern and *Step Two* in which you owned it by reciting the words in the previous chapter, you can now move on to *Step Three*. In this step, you will create a silent space into which you will surrender. Surrender is done at the level of body, not at the level of mind. To surrender is to silently observe, with detachment, what is going on at a physical level.

Here's how to do it:

- Find the physical sensation as it relates to the emotion that you identified in *Step Two* and explore it. Let's say for example, that you are feeling shame – you might notice that shame comes with an experience of rising heat in your body. You might notice the heat in your face and throat. You might also notice that there is a resistance to the experience and that your mind wants to run away. You might become aware of a cringing feeling in your body.
- Explore what you are feeling as it is occurring in the body (not the mind). Witness it with detachment as if it is occurring on a movie screen in 4D. You feel everything, but it is with the neutral gaze of

a scientist. You are more curious than concerned, less personal and more detached. Your mind might be chattering away; gently put the mind aside as you keep exploring what's happening in your body.

- Spend about 45 seconds to a minute doing this and then reflect on that exploration. Ask yourself: *What just happened in that space?*
- The answer will be one of three possibilities: *Shift, no-shift, or trap*, all of which I will describe in the next chapters.

That completes *Step Three*.

WHAT STEP THREE DOES

There is a yogi saying: "You can't get out of the mind using the mind."

Reflecting on the sequence of the pattern determines why this is so. Recall that by the time your mind becomes aware of the pattern, you've already taken action. Your conscious mind (the thought that completes the pattern) follows—it doesn't lead—and therefore, your thoughts will always support the pattern that is running. So how then are you to deconstruct a pattern? It stands to reason that through, is the only way out.

You cannot consciously "let go" of a pattern - you must *surrender*, and in the process of surrendering, the pattern gets deconstructed. When I say surrender, I don't mean for you to take the position of being a victim. To surrender at the level of action, behaviour or belief, is to give up. To surrender at the level of pattern, on the other hand, is the most powerful thing you can do. What happens in this space of surrender is you allow your conscious mind to catch up with what your subconscious has known all along: The pattern is providing a partial picture of the totality of your situation.

You surrender by letting go of your mind's way of perceiving, i.e., evaluating, comparing, labelling, resisting, striving, judging, so you can experience only your physical sensation. The act of surrender enables your subconscious to distinguish two separate realities arising simultaneously. The first reality is the reality as given by the pattern: The moment is contained in this pattern, and it is difficult to perceive the world in any other way. It is a reality as the pattern knows it.

Your body, on the other hand, is experiencing the situation through the changes in its vibration – a vibration that responds to the information streaming in through your senses. These two inevitably don't line up, and voila: Your brain lets that pattern go.

PITFALLS AND HOW TO AVOID THEM

Having taught this technique to many, I am aware of how readily people leap over this step. Surrender does not come naturally. We are taught to fix our problems; not to experience what is going on in our body as a result of them.

People often ask, does surrender mean that I have to accept the physical sensation? The answer is no. To *accept* is to expect the same response next time. Acceptance is equal to giving up.

Allowing is the *opposite* of giving up. To allow means to stand in the centre of the fire, feeling every lick of the flames with the courage to not turn away. As you surrender, you let go of the need or desire for your experience to be any different than it is. However, to do this, you must surrender at the *level of your body* and not at the level of your mind.

Recall that your body is always in the now which makes your experience—at least as far as the body is concerned—eternal and everlasting. To surrender at the level of the body is to align yourself with your body's way of perceiving. Your mind knows things will shift, but your body is simply present to *what is*. Surrendering into your body's experience allows you to be *a witness* to what is, just as it is. After all, there is nothing else for you to experience other than what is occurring at the moment. As far as your body is concerned, there is no other emotion and no other physical sensation than the ones you are having. Therefore, what is there to push away?

Without surrendering, your mind will keep intervening. Your mind's access to past and future means that it knows the present moment is temporary and that sooner or later, you will be experiencing a different emotion and a different physical sensation. Because your mind understands the world differently, it argues with your body, telling it that it shouldn't feel this way or that it doesn't have to feel this way. In so doing, it forces your body to remain steadfast. *There is nothing else*, your body argues back, and it roots itself deeper into the experience. In this way, a perpetual conflict arises between your body and your mind that keeps the pattern firmly in place. Without surrender, the witness, which resides in your subconscious and connects your mind and your body, is thoroughly occupied with this debate and has no way of observing the pattern for what it is: a partial picture derived from the past. Surrendering enables your brain to identify this and to let the pattern go, creating space for a new one to emerge.

SHIFT, NO-SHIFT OR TRAP

Having spent a minute or two in the space of surrender, the final part of *Step Three* is to invite your mind back in to assess what, if anything, occurred in that space. There are three possible outcomes: *Shift, no-shift, or trap.*

We will get to *shift* and *no-shift* in a moment. Let's first address *trap*.

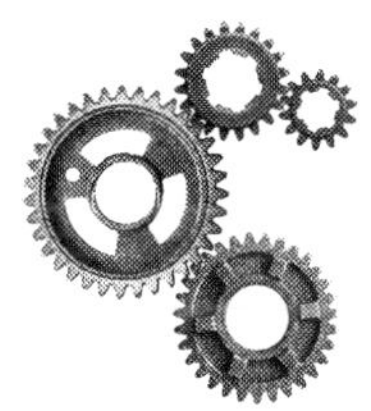

Chapter 9: Trapped in the Known

The 4-Step Repatterning Technique enables you to respond optimally at the moment. To do this, you need to be able to pull the optimal response from the totality of all possible responses. To make this possible, you first need to let go of the pattern that informs you that it already *knows* the "right," or best, response. In the space where that belief, behaviour or action once resided, you need to create a void.

It is not the opposite that you are seeking here (lying is bad vs lying is good) – what you need is best described as a *non-relationship* (the value of lying is contextual; lying is sometimes optimal depending on the situation, for example: "No sir, Anne Frank is not hiding in the attic").

Letting go of your patterns is the equivalent, therefore, of letting go of your convictions (your knowns) and yet, letting go of 'the known' is precisely what your existing pattern box is attempting to avoid. As your patterns are designed to keep you safe, they do not want you to spend any time in the unknown.

In efforts to protect you from the unknown, your mind has derived methods of side-stepping it. I call these the *four traps*.

Traps occur only in your mind. They are your mind's way of pulling you back into the safety of the box and thereby trapping you in your existing beliefs, behaviours and actions.

Traps are created alongside your patterns to hold them in place. Traps are not good or bad - they lock your patterns in place. Traps create the illusion that there is something real *inside* you that persists, which likewise creates the illusion that there is something *outside* of you that also persists. It is this belief in permanency that has you needing to do something with the pattern - to change it in some way. And the more you try to change it, the more you end up locking it in. I'll explain this phenomenon more as I get into the four traps in the discussion below.

The four traps are: *analysis, justification, catastrophizing and rebelling*.

Recall that at the end of *Step Three—Surrender*, you reflected on the minute in which you created the opportunity for surrendering, and you asked yourself the question: *What just happened in that space?*

The following description of the four traps will help you determine whether or not the answer is *TRAP*.

THE ANALYSIS TRAP

Analysis spins a self-centred world by telling you how things are or how they should be, based on a predisposition *given by your existing patterns*.

ANALYSIS = I MUST KNOW

Your mind believes that it can determine the correct course of action by analysing. It likes to mull things over and consider all of its various options before making a decision. This thinking appears productive, yet upon closer examination, you will find that all of this analysis always ends up supporting your prior conclusions. Why? Analysing is, of course, done by your existing patterns.

ANALYZING YOUR SENSATIONS AND BELIEFS

When Norah and I started working together, she believed that selling is pushy. As she started to deconstruct this pattern, the trap of analysis would move in to support her belief. In the space allowed for in *Step Three*, where surrender ought to be happening, Norah's thoughts would be exploring all the evidence for why selling is either pushy or not pushy. Sometimes the trap would find numerous examples where salespeople cajoled her into buying, and sometimes it would attempt to counteract itself by arguing the opposite: For example, *"selling isn't always pushy...remember when...."* Norah thought that this internal debate was a way of *counteracting* her beliefs, but in actuality, this flipping back and forth just *further supported* her belief that 'selling is pushy'.

Here is how analysis supports your existing beliefs. Perhaps you have heard the expression, "You can't see the forest for the trees." Norah started with the overarching belief, "Selling is pushy" (the forest). Now in efforts to counteract that belief, she looks for exceptions to the rule, "the time when the saleswoman suggested a more reasonably-priced item" (the tree). This exception, however, does not negate the initial belief; it is one exception to a rule that remains in place. No matter how many exceptions Norah found, selling continued to have a relationship to pushiness. It is that initial belief (selling is pushy) that needs to be deconstructed, and that can only happen by way of surrender.

ANALYZING YOUR EMOTIONS

When you judge your emotions or have thoughts about them, you are analysing them. It is not uncommon when I first start working with someone for them to respond to the question, "What are you feeling?" with what they are thinking. Feelings, so far as your mind is concerned, ought to be judged as appropriate or inappropriate. You ask, '*is it right to feel this way?*' or, you might investigate the origins of your experience: '*Why am I feeling this way?*'

Analysis can also have you compare how you feel in the moment with how you felt previously: '*I didn't always feel this way. I used to feel...*' If you can figure out your emotions, your mind tells you, then you can change them – you can make unpleasant ones go away. The problem with this assumption is that *thought is the last piece that completes a pattern*. Every thought you have is coming from *your box of patterns*. To analyse those thoughts, therefore, is to scramble inside that box in search of solutions that can only lead back to where you started. Again, you cannot get out of your mind using your mind.

INDICATORS

How do you know you're in the analysis trap? The following are indications:

1. **Comparison:** *I was feeling one way, and I am now feeling this way. Or, the feeling is now in my throat; it used to be in my chest.*
2. **Dismissing:** *I don't have to feel this way. It's alright, or, it doesn't matter.*

3. **Identifying:** *I know when I picked up this pattern – it started when I was very young. My mother was like this too.*
4. **Interpreting:** *I did it right, or, I did it wrong, Surrender worked, or surrender didn't work* -- **usually interpreted based on how you felt at the time of surrender. For example,** *I feel peaceful, so it worked,* **or,** *I feel angry, so it didn't.*
5. **Striving:** *I should be feeling positive, or, when I have deconstructed this pattern, I will feel a certain way.*

THE RESULT OF ANALYSIS

When you analyse, there are only two possible results available to you:

1. **Keep the pattern and continue to produce the same result in your life (as we know, analysing gets you back to where you started)**
2. **Strive for the exact opposite result, which will only result in the** *same* **outcome (since both are coming from inside the pattern)**

What analysis doesn`t show us is that both of these results exist within it.

An optimal pattern must contain neither of these results. After all, if the answer already existed within your pattern box, you would not have the problem. There is only one answer to the question, why? (As in *Why am I like this?* Or, *Why did she do that?* Or, *Why am I feeling this way?*) And the answer is: "Because it's a pattern."

Analysing is always a trap.

THE JUSTIFICATION TRAP

While analysis explores all possibilities, justification doesn't allow any room for doubt: This is the way it is, and there are no other options.

JUSTIFICATION = I KNOW

When you justify, you have a false sense that you are considering a reality – a real world out there that is defined by a certain truth. This truth appears to cut through the ambiguity of the situation you find yourself in, and so, therefore, it is accompanied by feelings of precision and certainty: *I must...*, or, *I should*. The justification trap is full of "shoulds" and "ought to's" while failing to accept life as it is. This trap does not question your so-called truth – instead, it only moves in to find evidence for it.

INDICATORS

When you are justifying, your statements will be peppered with the word "*because*." "*Because*" is this trap's operative word. '*I need to do this because*' or, '*I can't do that because*'. Sometimes the "because" is implied, but it's always lurking just beneath the surface.

If you can convince yourself that what you are feeling is correct and that it "makes sense" given your so-called "truth" about things, then the justification trap serves to strengthen your patterns: *I can continue to be angry because I am right. I must be embarrassed because my actions were wrong.*

Often this trap becomes defensive and will push back against any other opinions. Take, for example, this conversation with one of my workshop participants, Evelyn. Evelyn didn't own a car. Coming home required a subway ride and two buses to get to her daughter's daycare first, and then a third bus to get home. One day she told me she was particularly frazzled because, on top of her usual commute, she had to leave the house to get her hair done, which required she retrace her last two buses. Here was how the conversation went.

Me: *Why go to that hairdresser? Surely there is one close to work that you can go to at lunchtime.*

Evelyn: *Because I've gone to her for years. She's the only one I trust.*

Me: *So why not get the babysitter to pick up your daughter and you go directly to the hairdresser?*

Evelyn: *Because I have chicken in the fridge.*

Me: *Sorry?*

Evelyn: *I need to turn the chicken into a stew for my daughter's dinner. If I don't do it tonight, it will go off.*

Me: *So why not get the babysitter to do that?*

Evelyn: *Because she will not make it the way my daughter will eat it – she's very fussy.*

Me: *So why not give her a recipe?*

Evelyn: *Because she will use too much salt.*

Yes, I was triggering her trap. Luckily for her, she eventually saw it too. If your sentences are peppered with the word "because," then it is highly likely that you are caught up in the justification trap.

THE RESULT OF JUSTIFYING

Again, staying stuck in this trap only serves to reinforce the pattern that is already running. Nothing new gets created.

Justifying also often results in a divide between you and the people in your life because you can get defensive trying to protect your point of view – a point of view that is coming from the pattern.

Justifying is always a trap.

THE CATASTROPHIZING TRAP

In catastrophizing, your mind causes everything to be bigger and worse than it is. This trap triggers a lot of emotions. When caught in this trap, fear and panic can overwhelm you, anger can engulf you, and optimistic thinking can provide you with a way to avoid what is actually going on.

CATASTROPHIZING = I KNOW, AND IT'S BIG

There are two ways that this pattern plays out. First, it can make everything appear worse than it is. For example, Marie had a pattern that had her tolerating an unworkable relationship. Each time she entertained the decision to leave, the catastrophizing trap would move in, causing her to feel panicked: *I will be broke, lonely and miserable; I'm leaving my best friend.*

The other side of the catastrophizing trap is zeal. Ellen wanted her own business, but fear stopped her. When we explored her goals, the catastrophizing trap was immediately present: '*I see myself as a billionaire, on the stage in front of thousands. I own a yacht with a helicopter pad*', she would say.

The catastrophizing trap will tell you that great is better than good, millions are better than thousands, and that success is not a success unless it is over-the-top. In this case, the trap makes every small step you take appear irrelevant. *It is never good enough*, the catastrophizing trap informs.

Likewise the catastrophizing trap will spin you around with unnecessary worry -- the outcome will be disastrous, you can't possibly succeed, if you succeed your family will leave you, your boss will fire you, and the house will burn down.

INDICATORS

If you find yourself worried about disaster striking if you take a particular action, or if you find yourself telling yourself that your goals and what you're doing are never good enough, you are likely caught in a trap of catastrophizing.

THE RESULT OF CATASTROPHIZING

Both the negative and the positive sides of catastrophizing will keep you trapped in unworkable patterns. When you are overwhelmed by negative emotions, such as panic or fear, it is easier to remain in the pattern than to take action in another direction. Equally, when your vision of success is so grandiose, it is difficult to see how you can bridge the gap between here and there. The result is to stay rooted in the pattern rather than deconstructing it.

Catastrophizing is always a trap.

THE REBEL TRAP

This trap delivers a steady stream of, *you can't make me, and, F.U.* The rebel trap feels powerful. It is, therefore, the hardest trap to overcome.

REBEL = I KNOW THAT RULE IS WRONG

The interesting thing about the rebel trap is how automatically it defers to authority. Yes, I did say *defer*: Whether or not you choose to follow the rule or rebel against it, does not make any difference; either way, in this trap, *you believe that the authority has the power.* In other words, when you rebel, you do so precisely because you feel that you must follow all the rules. Underneath the rebel trap is a "good girl" or "good boy" who feels controlled by too many rules.

INDICATORS

The best indication of the rebel trap is an over-awareness of the rules and authority and a need to refute both. When caught in this trap, people make sweeping statements about "right" and "wrong," with authority and the rules always falling on the side of "wrong".

THE ROOT OF THE REBEL TRAP

Instead of dealing with the act of rebellion itself, you need to get under it to the pattern that leads you into rebelling.

To rebel is to accept that a power imbalance exists. When you rebel, you are like a fish in water that keeps trying to leap out and repeatedly lands right back in.

To stop the need to rebel, you must first understand that all rules are contextual. They work some of the time, in some situations. Consider the example I used earlier: "No, sir, Anne Frank is not hiding in the attic." If rules are contextual, how do you know which rule is right? The simple answer is, you can't. There is no way to tell which rule should be applied to which situation before the situation has arisen. Therefore, you need to catch the "should" before it arises: *I should? Says who? Which pattern?*

If rules are contextual, why rebel? Against what? The rule that you, yourself established, that says that rules are wrong? The authority that you have established inside, that now insists you mustn't follow the rules? To fight authority is to fight an illusion as if the illusion itself is real. The rebel trap creates the relationship to authority first, and then goes to war against that relationship, giving authority, even more sway over you.

So now there is another problem: You might be thinking, *Okay, if rules are contextual, then I can speed/I can eat what I want/I can have it my way* -- but that too is the rebel at play. *Who* is the "I" who wants their way? That "I" consists only of patterns, created in the past, held together by traps—the "I" fighting itself—and wanting its way against the authority, it put in place, to hold itself in place.

The only way to truly "rebel" is to deconstruct the pattern for authority. You need to be able to follow the rules or not follow the rules, without the need to make anything wrong in the process. A deconstructed pattern is no longer concerned with the principles of right and wrong. You become relaxed about rules, knowing you will respond optimally for each situation.

An optimal pattern will bend the rules when necessary, follow the rules when it is the optimal thing to do and break the rules if the rules bring harm to another. It is no longer one-size-fits-all, and this ability to bend and shape the rules to fit the situation means that, funnily enough, if a rebellious act is needed, you will be able to rebel, but you will do so, without the need to make anything wrong in the process.

As you bring more and more awareness to the rebel trap, and your traps in general, you will head naturally in this direction. There is openness to new experiences; an allowing that comes only from the fluidity of the moment. Learning to recognise the four traps is the key to making this possible.

THE RESULT OF THE REBEL TRAP

Of all of the traps, the rebel trap is the most difficult to manage. There are three reasons for this:

1. The rebel is the trap that you are most likely to confuse as being a part of your identity. "I am a rebel," you might say, and not without a certain level of pride. Identification makes it all the more difficult to see it as a trap and to catch it when you are caught up in it.
2. Unlike the catastrophizing trap that can cause you to feel disempowered, the rebel trap feels powerful - and power is intoxicating.
3. What the trap rebels against is an authority, and by authority, I mean anyone who tells you what to do; and unfortunately, that will include me and this technique.

Rebelling is always a trap.

BREAKING FREE FROM YOUR TRAPS

If you find yourself in one of the above traps at the end of *Step Three*:

- The first thing to do is to be aware that you are in a trap. Recognising rebelling, justification, catastrophizing and analysing as a trap is, in itself, liberating.
- Next, don't try to control the trap. Don't make it wrong. Instead, give it a label. Say, "Justification," for example, and then return your mind gently to the space of surrender. Labelling works because your mind is always searching for understanding. Remember: the trap is there because your mind is trying to avoid being in the unknown. Providing a label for the trap pauses your mind. It is no longer confused because you placed the experience into a category that it can understand.
- Remember also that nothing about your mind or body is ever *wrong*. Your mind understands the world by reducing it down into something manageable, and it does this, by labelling things. Don't fight this tendency. Let your mind experience your world in its way (labelling) as your body experiences in its way (feeling). Categorising your thoughts, let's you get back the body and the state of surrender.
- Once you've labelled which trap you are in, catastrophizing, analysing, justifying, or rebelling, return your mind to observing your body's physical experience—i.e., return to *Step Three*—and surrender again.

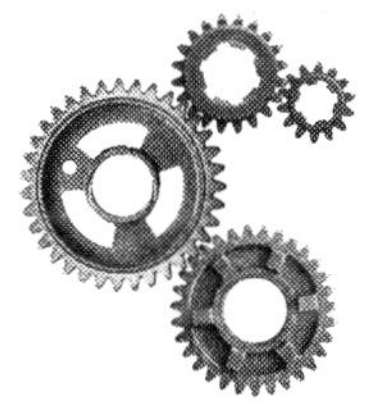

Chapter 10: Shift Or No-Shift

Besides trap, there are two other possible outcomes of *Step Three—Surrender*: shift or no-shift. I'll explain no-shift first.

NO-SHIFT

No-shift is easy to determine: nothing changes. In the space of surrender, everything remains the same. The physical sensation as it relates to the emotion is still present. You continue to feel the same emotion. There is no unexpected insight that brings a new perspective. You do not have any thoughts that lead you into one of the four traps I described in the last chapter.

If that is the case, label the experience "no-shift," and return to the space of surrender in *Step Three*.

You can also use "no-shift" when you drift off, which will likely happen when you first start this process. Instead of beating yourself up for drifting off and losing concentration, when you notice you have drifted, label what happened "no-shift," and return to the space of surrender. Be gentle with yourself and the drifting will stop.

SHIFT

The other possible outcome of *Step Three* is a shift: something changes. The physical sensation changes, the emotion changes, or a flash of insight occurs.

What feels distinctive about a shift is that it comes with an element of surprise: You were not anticipating the change that happened. Shift can be extremely subtle or quite dramatic, and either way is fine. It is not the *degree* of surprise that matters; it is the *unexpectedness* that counts.

Sometimes, in the space of surrender, you may feel the physical sensation melt away. Sometimes your body might take a deep breath that you didn't consciously try to take. Generally, a shift will bring with it a new, unexpected sensation.

Here is a list of possible shifts. Please don't limit yourself to these or strive to achieve these. Again, it is the element of surprise, no matter how subtle that is, that determines whether it is a shift or not.

- An unexpected deep breath
- A shudder
- Sitting up straight
- A surge of energy
- A smile
- Laughter
- The physical sensation dissolves
- Opening your eyes and everything looks brighter and more distinct
- Your body coughs
- An insight (a new thought that comes out of nowhere)

Again, this is just a list of possibilities. A shift is a highly-subjective experience that will be different every time.

Keep in mind that all *expected* outcomes are traps (namely, the analysis trap).

Note: Err on the side of caution when it comes to "insight." Recall that thought completes the sequence of a pattern. An insight can sometimes indicate the birth of a new pattern, in that the change in physical sensation and emotion went unnoticed until the moment a new thought arose, however, *this is unusual*. Typically, thought is an indication of a *trap*, rather than of a *shift*. That said, if the thought surprises you, bringing with it an unexpected insight, then it is okay to consider it a shift.

WHAT SHIFT DOES AND DOESN'T INDICATE

When you first start to go through the steps, you may find yourself striving for a shift mistakenly thinking that shift is an indication of a deconstructed pattern. Please don't do this. During the 4-Step process, there is no way to judge the outcome. The sole indicator that you have successfully deconstructed a pattern and replaced it with an optimal one is that you start getting different results you get in your life.

So what does shift indicate? It indicates one thing and one thing only: You are now running a different pattern. However, whether that pattern is a brand new pattern or just a different, already existing pattern that lives inside the box, remains undetermined.

Your goal, of course, is to remove the pattern altogether, creating a *void* in the pattern box which generates the necessary conditions for the birth of a new pattern. But—and it is an important but—the only way you can determine when that has happened is when you no longer take that action, adopt that behaviour or believe that belief. In other words, the only way to tell if you have done it correctly is when things change in your life, and you get different results.

For example, if you are applying the 4 Steps to your money patterns, then you'll know you have deconstructed the patterns when your bank account reflects such. Likewise, if you are applying the 4 Steps to your relationship, you'll know you have deconstructed the old pattern(s) when the relationship improves.

THE RESULT OF SURRENDER

When you surrender in *Step Three*, so much is accomplished: First, surrendering brings about a completely new body vibration. Recall that your body's vibration changes in response to its environment, which in turn alerts the subconscious to go off in search of a pattern that most closely aligns with the vibration. In the search for that pattern, the first place your body will turn to is your existing box of patterns (your existing box provides you with the quickest response time). As you surrender, you add an unexpected element to the experience which then alters your body's vibration and again triggers the search for a different pattern. Your subconscious dips back into the box, but this time there is no existing pattern that aligns with your body vibration, and so a brand new pattern is birthed.

But wait - is there a question bubbling up? Are you asking: *If that is what happens, then why can't I just add a new element to the situation, such as saying an affirmation or snapping an elastic band on my wrist? Why doesn't that work the same way?*

To understand the difference, we need to look at the difference between a pattern *interrupt* and a pattern *deconstruct*.

PATTERN INTERRUPT VERSUS PATTERN DECONSTRUCT

Pattern interrupts, such as the snap of an elastic band, will indeed cause a shift in your vibration and therefore do, in turn, trigger an internal need for a different pattern. However, pattern interrupts are a distraction *away* from the current situation and pattern, instead of being opportunities to *get closer* to the current situation and pattern. The snap of the elastic does change your body's vibration, but in a way that has you become *further* removed from what is going on in the moment.

Surrender is not a pattern interrupt; surrender does something much more powerful. Surrender slows down the sequence of the pattern and allows you to witness your body's vibration at a subconscious level. Here is where the two distinct realities arise simultaneously: the *actual* vibration of your body as given by the *actual* situation you are in and the *partial* reality given by the pattern that is running. And as mentioned, when those two don't line up, the pattern that is running collapses and the Pattern Maker in you creates a new one.

That is the power of surrender. It is only by allowing "*what is*" that your pattern will deconstruct and the birthing of a new pattern can happen. Any "resistance to the resistance" will lock in the pattern. Any analysis, justification, rebelling, or catastrophizing will cause the pattern to dig its heels in and stay put. It is only through *surrender* that your pattern and identity can shift from singular and fixed to a myriad of expression, which makes surrender the single most powerful thing you can do.

Surrendering is an art. It is the allowing of your body's experience *just as it is*. It recognises the unique way that your body relates to the moment as eternal and never-changing. When you surrender, you become witness to your body. Allow your mind to do what your mind does; your job is to keep coming back to the physical sensations and emotions of your body, observing them without judgment, and without connecting those physical sensations with those emotions or with that thought. As best you can, allow all three parts of the pattern to arise, independent of each other, and then observe fully, surrendering to what is occurring at a physical level.

Step Three marks a crucial juncture in your progress. This step is the heavy lifter in the 4 Step Repatterning Technique. I recommend that you spend at least two weeks applying Steps One, Two and Three, before advancing to Step Four.

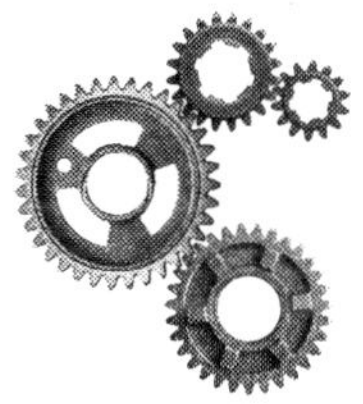

Chapter 11: Step Four - Trust

Now that you have identified the pattern you are running in *Step One*, have owned the pattern in *Step Two*, and have surrendered to your body's experience in *Step Three*, you are ready to move to the final step of the Repatterning technique: *Trust.*

To complete *Step Four*:

- Recite out loud: "I trust this moment to deliver the optimal pattern I need."
- Then pause for 15 seconds to connect with your body's experience.

That completes *Step Four*.

WHAT STEP FOUR DOES

To understand *Step Four*, you must first understand *what* you are trusting in when you say, "I trust this moment." What exactly do we mean by 'this moment' and what is it that you are putting your trust in?

WHAT IS IN THIS MOMENT

Three things are present at "this moment." The first is your vast-warehouse within (as defined below), the second is your goals and aspirations, and the third is other people. These three combined create the conditions for the birth of an optimal pattern in *Step Four*. Let's explore each in turn and then how they come together to support you.

#1: YOUR VAST WAREHOUSE WITHIN

The first thing that exists is everything that you have ever seen, heard, smelled, tasted and touched in your lifetime. Your subconscious mind is remarkable! It records *everything*; not only what you are aware of knowing, but also everything that you just happen-by, for example, the license plate on the car that passed you on the highway on the way to work. Of course, most data is completely superfluous, and so you mostly remain unconscious to it, as you should; however, it is there and available in your subconscious mind should you need it. I call this store-hose of information, the vast warehouse within.

Take a moment to consider what you just read in the above paragraph. You have housed, although not in a consciously-accessible format, every experience you have ever had. How much have you read, studied, overheard, seen, learned, as it relates to your area of concern? For example, if you are running an unworkable pattern in your relationship, how much information on love and relationships do you think you've come across in your entire lifetime? And, if you are like most people, as this problem persisted, the amount of effort that you put into looking for a solution also increased, and so you gathered even more data. All of that data, plus so much more, is housed in what I call *the vast warehouse within.*

#2: YOUR GOALS AND ASPIRATIONS

The second thing that exists within "this moment" is your goal, that which you are trying to achieve. Now, just a note on this. I know that there are times that you have conflicting desires and many personal development programs insist that this internal conflict is a detriment to your success. Please put that idea to the side. Your subconscious is aware of the global 'want' within, and it is this direction that the optimal pattern will move you in. Even if your goals are conflicted, the optimal pattern can take care of all of these internal conflicts and still lead you in the right direction for your success.

#3: OTHER PEOPLE

The third thing that exists in the present moment is whoever is being affected by the situation you're in: in other words, other people. "This moment" includes their goals, their desires, and what is best for them, as well as for you.

THE COMBINATION OF THESE THREE CAUSES THE OPTIMAL PATTERN

Now, let's put all of this together to understand what happens in *Step Four*. As you know, you cannot consciously determine what pattern is optimal for the moment because anything that you determine to be the "correct" pattern must already be an existing pattern from the box. So in this final step, all that remains for you to do is *trust*. Trust that the Pattern Maker in you—the part of you that is responsible for creating patterns—will create the optimal pattern you need.

That said, this trust is not blind trust. The optimal pattern results from your body vibration, and that vibration is the sum of everything that exists at that moment. This vibration includes the information coming in through your senses as it relates to the situation; the people who will be affected by any change in that situation; the direction that you and the group need to move in, and all of your past experiences that make up your vast warehouse. To recite, "I trust this moment to deliver the optimal pattern I need," is to trust in your subconscious to bring all of these elements together to bring about an optimal result.

An optimal pattern not only takes care of you, but it also takes care of those around you. Patterns pulled from the past are always self-centred, meaning the primary focus is always on you and your needs (either in a positive way or, in a negative way). Optimal patterns are different. Being aligned with the present situation and moment, they deliver a holistic result. It is no longer only about "you" and your needs; it becomes about "us" and our needs. The rest of the book explains this in detail. For now, let's complete Step Four before we get to the beauty of optimal patterns.

PITFALLS AND HOW TO AVOID THEM

You could argue that Step Four is redundant. After all, as soon as a pattern deconstructed, a new pattern was immediately birthed by your subconscious to take its place. You don't have to do anything to cause that to happen.

However, when you *trust*, you are doing something vital.

Deconstructing a pattern requires that you do something that every human being fears: to slip into the unknown. Please don't underestimate the enormity of this leap of faith. Your conscious mind has no way of causing a new pattern; as far as it is concerned, the old pattern is enough. Regardless of how courageous you may feel, deconstructing a pattern is still a lot to ask.

In *Step Four*, you respect the enormity of this leap and acknowledge your mind's bravery.

That completes the 4-Step Repatterning Technique.

For review, and so you can refer quickly to the technique, here are the 4 Steps in their entirety:

STEP ONE—IDENTIFY THE PATTERN

What is the:

- Physical Sensation?
- Emotion?
- Thought?

That completes *Step One*.

STEP TWO—OWN THE PATTERN

- **"I created the physical sensation, _______"** (name it), pause and experience this physical sensation in your body.
- **"I created the emotion, _______"** (name it), pause and experience this emotion in your body.
- **"I created the thought, _______"** (state it) and then notice where that thought lands in your body; there will be a physical response somewhere that results from this thought.
- Lastly, state, **"And because I created it, I can let it go."**

That completes *Step Two*.

STEP THREE—SURRENDER

Surrender by letting go of:

- Striving
- Resistance
- Judgment
- Evaluation
- Comparison

After approximately 30 to 45 seconds, reflect and ask yourself:

- Shift?
- No-Shift?
- Trap?

If Trap, label the Trap:

- Analysis
- Justification
- Catastrophizing
- Rebelling

And return to the space of surrender

If No-Shift

- Return to the space of surrender

Repeat a maximum of three times.

If Shift

- Continue to Step Four.

That completes *Step Three*.

STEP FOUR—TRUST

- Recite: "*I trust this moment to deliver the optimal pattern I need.*"
- Pause; experience your body for 10-15 seconds.

That completes *Step Four.*

If you have been following the recommended schedule, you are now at the four-week mark. From here on in, you will be using all four steps in the 4 Step Repatterning Technique. Over the next two weeks, you will start to experience real and lasting changes in your life. If that does not happen, it means that there is something that needs tweaking in your application of the technique.

If that's the case, contact us at www.AdeleSpraggon.com and book a free one-on-one coaching call. If you are applying the technique correctly, you will get results. If you are not getting results, something is off. Call us and we'll explore it together.

PART THREE:
The Pattern Maker Way

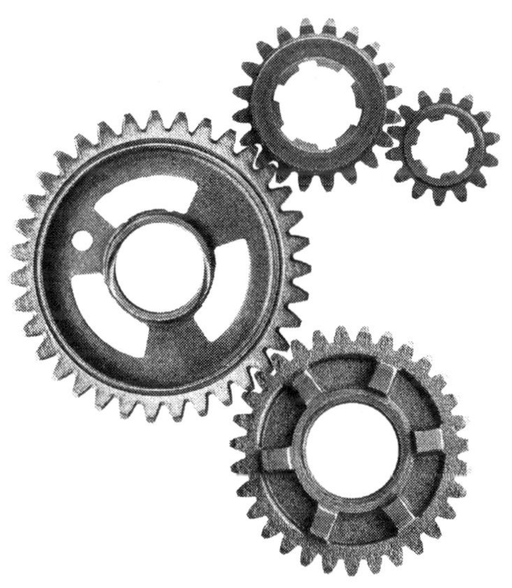

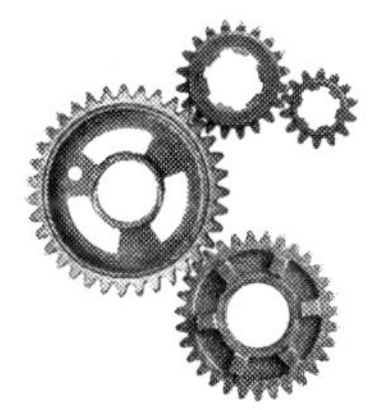

Chapter 12: Plasticity - Your Brain is Built to Rewire

Now that we've walked through the 4-Step Repatterning Technique together, I'd like to draw on some research and practices in the neuroscience field to help you understand why initially you will need six-weeks and patient application before you start to see results. I'll be using the research described in Norman Doidge's *The Brain's Way of Healing: Remarkable Discoveries from the Frontiers of Neuroplasticity*[2] to help with this understanding.

In his book, Doidge tells the story of a woman named Jan. Jan had a goal: She wanted to be pain-free, which is how she came to be sitting in Dr Michael Moskowitz's office listening carefully as he explained the workings of her brain. Jan suffered from chronic pain, and yet, as Dr Moskowitz was explaining, there was no longer any physical reason for the pain.

As with many chronic pain sufferers, Jan's body had since healed from her injury. When the injury first occurred, it, of course, required attention, and so her body and her brain worked together to protect that area of her body. At the time, Jan's brain, picking up on her body's distress, started firing the necessary pain messages signalling to Jan to slow down and be extra cautious for a while.

And then something went awry: Her body healed, but her brain failed to recognise that healing. What had started as acute pain (temporary) became chronic pain.

Dr Moskowitz also wanted Jan to be pain-free, which was why he took his time as he carefully explained to Jan how her brain was misfiring. To help with this goal, he used three drawings. The first drawing depicted the brain of a pain-free person. The second showed a brain correctly sending the necessary message of pain to an area of the body that was damaged. The third was of a brain incorrectly responding and thereby creating chronic pain.

Dr Moskowitz spent extra time on the third picture, showing Jan how her brain was escalating the experience of pain because it incorrectly believed the body needed additional attention and was trying its best to bring about healing. In doing so, it was knitting together more neurons into additional pain channels.

Dr Moskowitz explained to Jan that pain had now taken her brain hostage. Neuron channels that were meant to be available for other purposes were now hijacked by the pain, making it impossible for her to experience anything other.

For Jan and Dr Moskowitz to reach their mutually-shared goal of her being pain-free, she would have to hijack the areas of her brain *back* from the pain pathways. And he had just the tool to help her do it.

He handed her the three drawings. "The next time you experience pain," he instructed, "rather than pop a pill or in some other way distract yourself, turn inward, *toward* the pain, and picture the brain going through these three stages: from chronic pain to acute pain and finally, to no pain."

Jan embraced the technique with gusto. After all, what else was there for her to do? By then, the pain was so intense that she was spending upward of eight hours a day in a massage chair. Sitting, in that chair day after day gave her plenty of opportunities to do as the doctor ordered.

At first, progress was slow. In the first few weeks, she experienced momentary glimpses of being pain-free before the pain returned. Jan did not allow the setbacks to stop her and instead saw them as a positive sign that urged her on.

Then at the six-week mark, she was remarkably rewarded. Having followed the instructions diligently, she suddenly became pain-free.

Dr Moskowitz was impressed. Scanning her brain, he discovered the reason for this remarkable success: Each time Jan had done the activity, the neurons that had knitted together to bring the experience of pain, weakened. At first, the weakening was barely perceptible, with only momentary glimpses of what it would be like without pain - until, that is, the six-week mark. At that point the neurons had weakened to the point that they pulled apart and snapped together into different channels, leaving Jan completely free of pain.

Dr Moskowitz now specialises in chronic pain. Some of his patients have similar experiences to Jan's and reach their goal of being pain-free. Others don't. Why?

It turns out there are two ways that Dr Moskowitz's patients approach the visualisation activity. Some, like Jan, take on the role of being active participants in their healing. They follow the instructions as designed, they trust him as their doctor, and they expect their healing to take time. Others follow the instructions in *anticipation* of becoming pain-free.

Can you guess which group is typically able to sustain the technique for the length of time it takes to weaken the neurons? The patients with an expectation of reward give up long before the technique can work its magic. "Nothing's happening," they say. "This doesn't work." Six weeks, inside an expectation of reward, is a long time to stick with something.

The patients who stick with the technique for six weeks, however, go on to achieve remarkable results.

Now, let's compare what Dr Moskowitz does with his patients to the 4-Step Repatterning Technique. You just started applying the 4-Step Repatterning Technique to an area of concern in your life. Like Dr Moskowitz's patients, you will have momentary glimpses that will urge you on, but lasting results will take time. Why is that?

Although it has yet to be proven through brain scans, I think it is safe to assume that your pattern—the one that is resulting in the unwanted behaviour, belief or action—is the result of neurons that are knitted together to create a particular channel in the brain. Just like Jan's chronic pain, this knitting together limits the physical sensations, emotions, and thoughts available to that area of the brain. It can, therefore, be said, in much the same way that Dr Moskowitz explained, that this pattern hijacks away from that area of your brain the capacity for you to experience anything other than the pattern's perspective.

Moreover, when going through the technique, you turn inward (*Step One*). Dr Moskowitz's patients are also instructed to turn toward the pain instead of *away* from it. Instead of distracting themselves using pills or other avoidance techniques, they use the pain as an opportunity to apply the method prescribed.

When you use the technique, you, too, use your pain (in this case the emotional pain that comes in the form of "something is wrong" messages experienced as self-doubt, fears, *I'm not good enough* thoughts, upsets, annoyances, irritations, and so on) as an indication that you are running a less-than-optimal pattern. And similarly, instead of distracting yourself using techniques such as affirmations, breathing exercises, positive thinking, and others, you to turn *toward* the pattern and identify your physical sensation(s), emotion(s) and thought(s).

Finally, the key to Dr Moskowitz technique is the patient's active participation in their cure. Active participation comes in the form of the patient's willingness to accept that their brain is responsible for creating the unnecessary pain signals. Typically, people *manage* their pain; but when one manages their pain, they become victim to it. With Dr Moskowitz's technique, the patient first needs to understand that *their brain* is creating the pain and that that pain is no longer necessary. Positioning themselves as the creator of the pain puts them back in control of it. Pain is experienced, yes; but because the pain is unnecessary; it is something that can now be released.

So, too, does the 4-Step Repatterning Technique invite ownership. Instead of being a passive bystander of circumstances that seem beyond your control, you acknowledge your active participation in the making of the pattern. "I created that," you state firmly in *Step Two*, "and because I created it, I can let it go." This statement, when coupled with an understanding of how patterns work, flips the switch. Like Dr Moskowitz's patients, you don't own the *result* of the pattern (in the case of his patients, the result is the pain *itself*, in your case, the result equals the action, behaviour or belief that is taken by the pattern); instead, you own the pattern itself, putting you back in a position of control.

The result of applying the 4 Step Repatterning Technique results in a similar experience to what Jan had when she teased apart the neurons in her brain that were causing her chronic pain. In your case, however, rather than chronic pain, what you experience is the limited understanding that your current pattern allows.

This current channel in the brain, (the one that makes up this pattern), will initially take time to tease apart, for the sole reason that like Jan's pain, the pattern is now chronic. Once your brain knows how to rewire; however, it will no longer take six-weeks to get results. This initial six-week window is because your brain is not familiar with Repatterning. Once it is, it catches on pretty quick, and the experience of Repatterning gets easier and easier.

But now, as we move onto Step Three, the comparison of the 4-Step Repatterning technique to Dr Moskowitz's method ends. Where Dr Moskowitz's technique and the one you learned about in this book differ is that his patients know the desired outcome—to be pain-free—and his visualisation technique moves them steadily toward that outcome. "Imagine your brain like this one," he instructs, showing them a brain that is without pain.

But what is the only thing that you can know with absolute certainty when it comes to deconstructing a pattern? The only thing that you can know for sure is that *you don't know* how to achieve your objective. Yes, you know that you don't want the current result that the pattern is providing you—i.e., the current action, behaviour or belief that the pattern delivers—but that is all you can know. Unlike Dr Moskowitz's patients, you cannot determine your goal as being the opposite of the experience the pattern is giving you. And this means that, unlike Dr Moskowitz's patients, you cannot use visualisation to imagine the outcome. Recall that the pattern is already aware of both itself and the opposite of itself, and therefore you already know that the opposite of itself is not the optimal goal. So then what is?

Well, that remains a mystery throughout the 4-Step technique. Therefore, in place of visualisations, willpower, commitments, mindset techniques, and so on, the element of surrender (*Step Three*) is added. When you surrender at this point in the technique, you give up all thought that you can know what the desired outcome is, and you allow the optimal pattern room to deliver the optimal results for the situation.

With each application of the four steps, the neuron pathways that connect that pattern and deliver a limited result weaken, until eventually, they snap apart, connecting themselves to different neurons and creating brand new patterns.

THE PLACEBO EFFECT

As Doidge explains in his book, in the early days of Dr Moskowitz's research, he wondered if his patients were experiencing a placebo effect. A well-known example of a placebo is a sugar pill: The sugar pill is not actual medicine, and yet the patient's belief that the pill will cure them is enough to bring about a cure. Placebos have a real, measured effect on the brain and, therefore, should not be underestimated. However, as Dr Moskowitz points out, the issue with placebo effects is they don't last long. Some consider hypnosis a placebo because it quickly changes the sequence of thoughts in the brain, enabling someone to think and feel differently relatively quickly. But although hypnosis eliminates pain in chronic pain patients, the effects don't usually last more than a week or two.

To fully reprogram the brain, takes time. Dr Moskowitz's technique was not a placebo cure. Six weeks was, and is, required for the desired change to take place for the long term.

Repatterning is also not a placebo. It too takes time, and conscious effort, particularly as you first start working the technique. So please put aside the expectation of instant results and give Repatterning the six weeks required for the brain to become used to creating new pathways.

Once your brain gets used to this technique, it won't always take six-weeks to create new patterns. With consistent application, you will find that the Repatterning process speeds up and in time you will be shifting patterns in a matter of days, then in just a few applications, and then continuously, every time you apply the Four Steps. To begin, please be patient as your brain learns to respond to the technique.

A BRAIN DIVIDED: A NEW LOOK AT YOUR BRAIN

WHY DO WE NEED THE UNKNOWN?

For the duration of this book so far, I have been referring to the different parts of the brain that are involved in the 4-Step Repatterning Technique as the *conscious* and the *subconscious* parts of the brain. A book called, *The Master and His Emissary: The Divided Brain and the Making of the Western World* [3], by Dr Iain McGilchrist, provides another lens through which to interpret why and how the 4-Step Repatterning Technique works.

Dr McGilchrist suggests that as human beings, we don't have one brain, but that, in effect, we have *two*. He states that our divided brain has a left and right hemispheres, each of which plays a different role.

According to Dr McGilchrist, the right hemisphere takes a holistic account of the world around you. It is your sentry, remaining vigilant and alert to potential predators and mates that might be nearby. In this role, it is on constant alert, always drinking in the totality of your environment indiscriminately, without judging or evaluating what it is absorbing.

A DEEPER LOOK AT OPTIMAL PATTERNS

This hemisphere is what I call *body wisdom*. It is responsible for the absorption of all of the information stored in your vast warehouse within. It is where the awareness of your body vibration occurs and is what makes available the holistic perspective you tap into when you are creating optimal patterns.

The role of the left hemisphere—what I term *mind wisdom*—is to prioritise that which is previously known. Mind wisdom is the conscious part of your brain. Its principal concern is utility, and its primary function is to turn the world into a resource for its own use. To do this, it seeks out the familiar.

In his book, Dr McGilchrist explains the difference between the two hemispheres in this way: Imagine a bird trying to extract a seed from the ground, and the ground is covered in pebbles. To accomplish this task, the bird uses its left hemisphere to provide it with a narrow, focused span of attention on something it already knows. Meanwhile, its right hemisphere is engaged in a very different task: that of being broadly vigilant for opportunities and threats that could come from anywhere.

Dr McGilchrist explains that for you to operate in this world, your right and left hemispheres must see the world through different lenses. Your right hemisphere cannot discriminate; it must be open to whatever is, and it must drink in the whole and not the parts. It is alert to what is going on in the moment and be unconcerned with the past or the future.

Your left hemisphere, on the other hand, is always dividing things into parts. It must categorise, label, sort, judge and evaluate, reducing as much as it can into things and information that can be manipulated and utilised based on prior knowledge.

It is your right hemisphere that forms the connection to your body. The drinking in of your surroundings indiscriminately enables the totality of your experiences to be housed within you. However, to manipulate this data, you need to call on the wisdom of your left brain. Your left hemisphere can explicate. It turns the raw material gathered by your right brain into something known and meaningful.

So your left and right hemispheres deliver different perspectives, and they need to. These different perspectives are why Dr McGilchrist and other neuroscientists have theorised that humans have two "brains," each playing remarkably different roles.

How does Dr McGilchrist's research relate to the sequence of a pattern? Although this is a very simplified understanding (I am no neuroscientist), I believe—and this is strictly my own belief—that your right hemisphere is where the first alert, or the stimulus, happens. As information streams in through your senses, your right brain is first alerted that a change in pattern is required. Communication then crosses from right to left, where the left hemisphere filters the holistic perspective gathered by your right brain into something manageable that it can work with - i.e., it activates the search for a pattern.

Although language requires both hemispheres, the ability to articulate using words is a left-brain tool. As Dr McGilchrist explains, words help us to represent (re-presence) our world by replacing individuality and the disordered with concepts.

Years ago, I had a personal experience that demonstrated to me what Dr McGilchrist means by this. On that particular day, I was doing walking meditation in a park. As I was walking and meditating, a black squirrel ran across the path in front of me.

In my meditative state, the language centres of my brain must have quietened because suddenly I was seeing "squirrel" for the very first time. With startling realisation, I recognised that I had never seen an actual squirrel before. What I had seen up until this point, were my labels of "squirrel," my learnings about squirrels and my memories of past squirrels, all of which had congealed in my mind into an impression of squirrel that was consistently overriding each individual squirrel that crossed my path. My left hemisphere was re-presencing squirrel for me each time I looked at a squirrel.

As I look back now, I know what must have happened: Somehow—and this was well-before my knowledge of Repatterning—I had deconstructed a pattern that up until then had brought me an experience that I was calling "squirrel." Before this experience, all of my encounters with squirrels had been filtered through my past. In other words, every situation I was in was never the actual situation I was in; my brain was creating a world that was arising out of patterns.

It might be easier to understand this concept by considering how children are in the world. To children, every experience is brand new. They don't see the world through filters; they see it with a luminosity of newness that fades over time as they create their pattern box.

Dr McGilchrist echoes my sentiments that there are inherent limitations inside of the way the conscious mind, or left brain, operates. The left hemisphere helps us to conceptualise the world around us, providing us with a means of manoeuvring through this world. However, as advantageous as this is, it has its limitations, especially when the patterns we have created deceive us.

Deception, you say? Yes. Consider the left brain phenomenon, called confabulation. Confabulation is a fancy term meaning, *to make stuff up*. Confabulation explains why your friend will look you directly in the eye and honestly tell you that her partner never takes her on a date when in the same moment, you can recall three dates that she and her partner have been on together in the last month. She is not lying when she says this; she has a belief (formed out of a pattern) that has replaced what is *actually* happening with *her beliefs about* what is happening.

And as much as you can see this all-too-often in the people around you, it helps to bear in mind that you are doing this to yourself all the time as well. Your left hemisphere is adept at making up stories to fit its already existing points of view.

However, according to Dr McGilchrist, over centuries of evolution, the left brain has positioned itself as the superior of the hemispheres. It is not superior, in reality. As Dr McGilchrist states, the right is the master and the left ought to be its messenger; however, we can most certainly see the effects of left over right all around us. To pick up from a conversation we started together in *Part One* of this book, positioning mind over matter has created a world that sees resources in terms of monetary value, that turns relationships into utilities, and that is convinced that rational thinking is superior to emotions. Accepting that our patterns make things up allows us to start questioning all of this.

If, for example, you said to your friend, "But that's not true: You two have been on three dates that I can think of in the last month." What do you suppose your friend would say?

I imagine the words you would hear would be something like, "Yeah, but that doesn't count", (imagine a dismissive tone here). "That was because...," and insert any excuse that allows your friend to perceive the three dates as the exception and not the rule, for example, "it was my birthday month; my mother is in Holland this month; the kids are acting up this month," thus supporting her belief and allowing her to keep the existing pattern in place.

Freedom comes when we can interpret the information given to us by our right brain (sensations, and "Something is wrong here") as an indication that we need to align our pattern. When we give up the idea that we can know the truth and instead start observing how our patterns continuously defend their singular perspective, then we can listen to the wisdom that our bodies and sensations hold. We can go into these body sensations, instead of running away from them, and we can change our patterns, thereby changing our brains.

Not being able to know the truth is freeing. An analysis is a heck of a lot of work, with very little reward. So let's turn to the 4 Steps to see how they support both the left hemisphere's need to know and the right hemisphere's ability to see beyond the current pattern.

Here is an illustration of the 4 Steps to help us out:

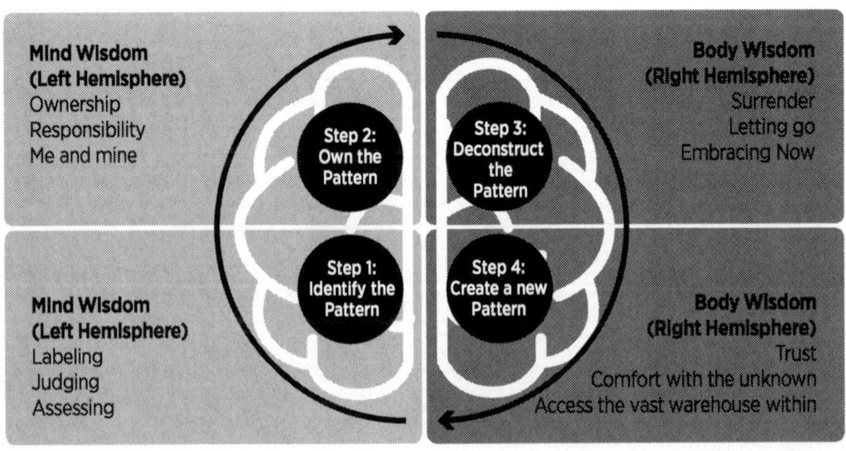

Recall that in *Step One*, you draw on left hemisphere wisdom, or mind wisdom. Your left hemisphere helps you to pin things down when the need to be precise arises. In efforts to help with this precision, it puts things into categories which helps you to comprehend the data. You capture your experience in language, giving you the necessary distance from the situation to both observe it and work with it.

Identifying the pattern, therefore, has the effect of freezing your physical sensation, emotion and thought for a moment, in much the same way that the label "squirrel" re-presenced the individual squirrel as it passed in front of my path and gave me a context for understanding. Your left brain provides you with a simplified version of reality; a simplification that you can use to override the vastness of your experience in much the same way that you would use a map when you are trying to plan a journey. Identifying the pattern becomes your map.

Step Two also uses your left hemisphere. *Step Two* acknowledges your mind's role as the creator of the pattern. It is the left that reduces your situations down into something knowable and something familiar. "I created that," you state emphatically in this step, confessing that this simplified version of the whole, your pattern, is of your own making. Your left brain has no access to the totality of the moment; it only has access to what it perceives based on its limited understanding. When you own the pattern, you take this into account.

In *Step Three*, you take a step to the right. Before looking at what is happening in Step Three through the lens of Dr McGilchrist's research, here is a paragraph from his book:

"Because the right hemisphere sees things as they are, things are constantly new for it ... [and therefore] it cannot have the certainty of knowledge that comes from being able to fix things and isolate them. In order to remain true to what is, it doesn't form abstractions and categories based on abstractions, which is the strength of denotative language. By contrast, the right hemisphere's interest in language lies in all the things that help to take it beyond the limiting effects of denotation and connotation: it acknowledges the importance of ambiguity. It, therefore, is virtually silent, relatively shifting and uncertain, where the left hemisphere, by contrast, may be unreasonably, or even stubbornly, convinced of its own correctness." (p. 80)

Step Three lives in ambiguity and uncertainty. As you move to *Step Three—Surrender*, you do so by letting go of your left brain's certainties. The only way to do this is by way of surrender: You witness, without judgment (judgment being a left-brain tool). Likewise, you must let go of comparisons, likes and dislikes, linear consideration ("This came before that"), analysis, justifications, catastrophizing ("This is worse," "That is better") and rebelling ("I can't," "You can't make me") and in place of all of this, you create an opening in which your right hemisphere can go to work.

And what is happening in that space of surrender? The holistic perspective of your right hemisphere and its ability to see things as they actually are is juxtaposed against the abstract world that gets re-presented by your left hemisphere. And in your gentle observation, your subconscious sees the misalignment between the two, the pattern deconstructs, and a new pattern takes its place. That new pattern is birthed from the totality of the moment as shown to you by your right hemisphere.

After about a minute or so of surrender, you again invite your left brain to re-presence for your right brain what occurred in that space. "Shift, no-shift, or trap?" you ask, bidding your left brain to do what it does best: categorise, label and act as the messenger on behalf of your right brain. This vital role is not just beneficial to your right brain; it is also a way to acknowledge again your left brain's role in the back-and-forth between the two that occurs within the 4-Steps. "Shift," it responds, or, "No-shift," it determines, and having done its job, it now relaxes again.

Of course, it doesn't always go that smoothly, and sometimes your left hemisphere continues to impress its pattern on your experience, and you get caught up in one of its four traps of justification, analysis, catastrophizing or rebelling. When this is the case, don't make anything wrong. Labelling the trap is enough to pause the experience so you can get back into your right brain and back to the task at hand.

Step Four—Trust, is solely the work of your right brain, as it should be. It is your right brain that is aware of the present moment and is, therefore, able to take into account the totality of your situation. Your right is not interested in the either/or of the pattern box. It sees things holistically and has no problem with paradox, and therefore, it provides the greatest opportunity for the optimal pattern to emerge.

Your right is also able to take context into account. It is concerned with the impact that your actions have on the whole and other people. To your right brain, your ego does not take precedence over others. From a holistic perspective, you are no more or less significant than anyone else.

And so in this final step, you allow the right brain to have the final say.

It is clear, then, that one of the major reasons the 4-Step Repatterning Technique works is it rebuilds the communication between the two hemispheres of your brain.

As Dr McGilchrist points out, throughout evolution, our brains have evolved to limit interaction between the left and the right. The left lacks the balanced understanding that the right provides, and frankly, has been wreaking havoc on our environment because of its emphasis on utility over relationships, and on thought and rationalisation over sensory experience.

Rebuilding this communication pathway within you and putting your right and left brains back into their respectful places is one of the benefits of the 4 Steps. Just how beneficial this is will be explored in the next chapters.

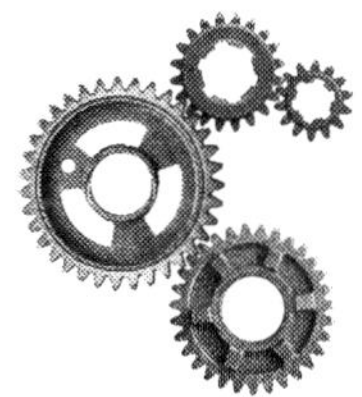

Chapter 13: Who Are You?

We stood on the roof of the small observatory looking out at the sea of stars above us. The astronomer leading the tour was explaining the night sky. "Do you know what you would see if you had a large enough telescope?" he asked.

I didn't.

"The curvature of space will bring you back to where you are, with you standing in this very spot, looking out from the roof of this observatory into space. With a large enough telescope, what you will see, will be the back of your own head."

What a great metaphor for patterns.

"How strong is your "I"? I asked a group of my workshop participants one day. "Who wants to find out?"

I divided them up into groups of two. "Choose who's going first. Ready? Okay – you have two minutes on the clock. Here's the exercise. You can talk about any subject that you want with one stipulation: You can't use the word "I."

"Easy," they said. "No problem."

That is, until about twenty seconds in. Laughter and giggles could be heard around the room. There were looks of confusion, long pauses and a chorus of "umms," as one woman piped up, "Can I say 'me'?" after which an explosion of laughter followed.

What is this identity? Who is this "I" that we refer to all the time?

Throughout history, we have come up with a variety of answers to this question. Philosophers, psychiatrists, scientists and religions have all put forth their theories, some of which are quite elaborate. All one needs to do is look at Sigmund Freud's theories on the Ego, the Id and the Superego to see just how elaborate these theories can get.

Could the answer be simpler than we have made it seem?

It is true that at first glance, it appears difficult to explain the inconsistency of our nature. It is easier to define a human being as a shape-shifter than as a singular identity because we are so readily shaped by our environment and our situations, making us appear complex. It is now known, for example, that depending on the environment we are in, we adopt different personalities. So distinctive are these different personalities that not only do our actions change, but so do our faces, the way we walk, what we say, the speed of our actions, and our posture. Human beings are so adaptable in fact, that some of our "sub-personalities" are strong enough to sign documents in their own distinct signature. No wonder we struggle to define the "I."

As we seek consistency within this "I," Freud's elaborate theories start to make sense. How else do we explain when we behave "out of character?"

Surely there must be a subconscious shadow that lurks within?

"Who are you?" I inquired of Valerie, one of the participants at the workshop. Valerie had joined the workshop to transform her business.

"Well...," she answered slowly, pondering her answer while speaking the words, "I guess I would have to say I am a mother, a wife, an image consultant...."

I gently interrupted her: "And if you'd never gotten married, had never had kids, and had chosen a different career, would you cease to be you?"

"Well...no," Valerie answered.

"So, who are you?" I nudged again.

"I would have to say I am a nice person. People say I am optimistic. I'm also a bit of an introvert."

"Are you always nice, optimistic and introverted? Are there times that you are mean, pessimistic or outgoing?"

"Sure, I guess...." I heard the confusion in Valerie's voice. "Then I don't know," she stated.

"Close your eyes," I suggested. "Tell me who you are right now, at this moment." I then encouraged her by saying, "I promise you there is a very real answer to this question, and when you get it, you will be liberated. Understand this and nothing will ever stop you again. You will never feel disempowered, no matter what the situation."

Valerie closed her eyes. "Right now, at this moment, I am curious", she said, "and I am seeking an answer to your question," she continued.

"And what are the physical sensations that are present inside 'curiosity' and the questions you are asking yourself?" I prodded.

"Well, I feel a little heavy," she said. "And there's a buzzy feeling in my forehead."

"And what is that?" I inquired. "What is the experience of 'heavy, buzzing, curious, and seeking'?"

"It's a pattern," she responded.

"Correct," I said. "So what does that make you?"

"A pattern?" she asked. A question mark hung in the air. "All I am is patterns?" she inquired further.

"No, not quite," I responded. "At this moment, all you are is this pattern. In a minute from now, you will be a different pattern. At the beginning of this session, you were a different pattern. But right now, at this moment, this is all you are. One pattern. *This* one pattern, to be exact." I paused for a moment. "How does it feel to be just a pattern, Valerie?"

As you enter the world of patterns, you enter the world of paradox. Much like the river that can be seen through one lens as being consistent and through another lens as never being the same twice, you, too, are in any given moment, only one pattern. When all of your patterns are strung together, there is a flow that you call "I."

"Sad!" she said emphatically. "That's so depressing. What about the soul? What about God?"

I smiled - I had heard this reaction before. In fact, I have yet to have anyone say to me, "You mean all I am is this pattern?! That's amazing! That's incredible! Wow." And yet I hope that by the end of this chapter this is exactly what you will be saying because, as I hope to demonstrate, patterns provide a richness and freedom beyond measure.

"How about we get back to God and soul in a moment," I suggested. "Before we go there, please tell me: How many physical sensations do you think the human being is capable of experiencing?"

Valerie thought for a moment, "Oh, I don't know," she said. "How about 500?"

"Alright," I said. "500 it is. And how many emotions?"

"Hmm...200?" she inquired.

"Sounds good to me," I said. "200 it is. How about thoughts? How many thoughts do you think we humans can have?"

"Ooh, that's a lot. Didn't you say before that we have about 40,000 thoughts a day? Let's go with 40,000."

"Done," I said. Whatever number Valerie had determined would have sufficed: even had she said as little as 100 in each category, the result would be the same, and so I continued. "So we have 500 physical sensations, 200 emotions and 40,000 thoughts. Now: How many combinations of these can we make?"

"Now that's a lot," Valerie said. "I wouldn't even know how to count that high."

"I think the answer you're looking for is *limitless.* There is an infinite number of combinations you can make out of a trinary system of 500 physical sensations, 200 emotions and 40,000 thoughts, wouldn't you say?"

"Yes...?" Valerie's voice trailed off into a question, still not sure where we were going.

"Do you know that the computer results from a binary system of one and zero? Think about that for a moment. A binary system of two digits has been used to create the internet, artificial intelligence, 3D printers...." I paused. "And here we sit Valerie, with a trinary system comprised of 500 physical sensations, 200 emotions and 40,000 thoughts and do you know what we say? What I typically hear is: 'I'm not enough. There's something wrong with me. I'm not smart enough. I can't do that. God, please help me'. Do you know what I imagine God's response is to that request?" Before she could answer, I answered for her, "*Oh for My sake, people, use what I gave you!*"

Valerie laughed. "I get it, she said, excitement growing in her voice. "With patterns, I can be anything! I just have to stop fixing myself and instead just let go of any pattern that isn't working!"

The understanding that no matter what you face is just a pattern brings with it a fully empowered view of yourself. There is nothing to fix, nothing to change and nothing to unearth in efforts to understand.

Remember that there are two different ways for you to experience your identity, each given by its respective hemisphere. What's important to keep in mind is that both are equally correct. According to your right brain's perspective, you are, like all living things, in a constant state of evolution. You are always arriving, never fixed and therefore, always unknowable. According to your left hemisphere's perspective, you are a series of patterns, each one of which is arising independently from the one that came before and the one that will follow. Each of these sub-identities stands alone and has no memory or understanding of the one that came before or the one that will follow. Each of your patterns has its own history, its own view of the future, its own values and ways of being in the world, and its own understanding of right and wrong.

We can illustrate the difference between these two perspectives using the metaphor of time. From the perspective of the left hemisphere, time is a series of incremental seconds, and each tick is separate from the one that came before and the one that will follow. As the minute hand moves, it does so after pausing momentarily in one place before advancing to the next.

Time seen by the right hemisphere occurs as a flow that has no beginning and no end. It is fluid motion; a process of sorts that cannot be pinned down.

It is the right brain's perspective that philosophers and psychiatrists have been using as a basis for understanding identity. In this hemisphere, the identity is never static and is therefore unknowable. It is specifically because of this that all theories about identity tend to be remarkably complicated.

So let us look: Are you an evolution – a continuous flow that moves through time? Yes, of course, you are. Are you equally able to see yourself as a collection of patterns, each one divisible from the one that came before and the one that will come next? Yes, of course, you can. Each perspective is valid, and each has its advantages and disadvantages. However, when you are confronted with an action, behaviour, or belief that is unworkable, then, "It's just a pattern" provides you with a huge advantage.

All you need to think about when it comes to your identity is this: Is the "I" that is arising, causing conflict around you? If so, let it go. Is the pattern not taking the actions that you need to take to get you to your goals? If so, then let it go.

It is, after all, *only a pattern*. And you have within you an infinite number of possible combinations of sensations, emotions and thoughts. In the absence of any one pattern, a new pattern will immediately be generated, and that new pattern will congeal, for a little while anyway, into a new "I", and you will arise again...and then again... and yet again.

Entering the world of acknowledging yourself as a Pattern Maker, will allow you to recognise the flimsy, insubstantial nature of your "I." Turning to look inward, you can see only physical sensations, emotions and thoughts and how fleeting and flimsy each one of these three parts of you is.

"It's just a pattern," Valerie laughed. "It's just a pattern, Adele! There's nothing wrong with me!"

That's right Valerie – and there has never been anything wrong with you. You are a miracle of creation. You are a Pattern Maker.

And this is the nature of transformation. You are a transformational genius, or at least you can be one, considering the trinary system that comprises you. Practice the 4-Step Repatterning Technique, and you will soon become adept at stepping out of one identity and into another, not once in a while, but continuously. As you do that, you enter the flow of life, where the newness of every moment carries you effortlessly forward.

What does life look like in the unknown? There are definite advantages. I want to share two stories with you to demonstrate some of these advantages.

AUBREY

Aubrey lived by her calendar, rigidly controlling, and being controlled by time. If anyone accidentally missed an appointment with Aubrey, it was viewed as a betrayal, and it was highly unlikely he or she would get a second chance.

This level of control also extended to money. Aubrey had very little freedom around money due to a strongly held belief that money was the root of all evil. She came by this belief honestly, having grown up in a well-to-do family that placed high expectations on the financial reward at the expense of emotional happiness.

Aubrey's transformation was dramatic. I don't mean dramatic in terms of results, because so long as you understand the 4 Steps and persistently apply them, you, too, can have these results over time; it was the speed of her results that made even my head spin.

Aubrey took on the 4 Steps with gusto. She already had a well-formed habit of sticking to her commitments, born out of her longstanding relationship to her calendar, and that now worked in her favour as she learned how to deconstruct her patterns.

Within a few weeks, I watched as Aubrey transformed before my eyes. Her life became one of spontaneity and fun. "I'm in Costa Rica. I've just been offered a job," she would laugh into the phone. Or she'd tell me, "I need to postpone our call – I've got a radio interview this afternoon," with excitement in her voice. Or once she said, "I just got a tattoo – I'll send you a pic."

Just weeks after starting to use the technique, people began to flock to her, drawn to her because they wanted what she had: ease and joy are enticing. As her life became rich, so did she. She took advantage of her gift of teaching and combined it with her love of travel by applying for and getting a job teaching in Dubai. She was singularly selected out of a pool of over 500 applicants.

Transformation on this level can only be achieved by stepping out of one identity and into another. Aubrey had tried to navigate around her controlling patterns, to no avail. Trapped inside her old identity, she would have been forever a slave to her calendar and money. Where change takes effort, transformation brings ease, and quickly.

LIANA

Liana lived a life of people-pleasing. She tried to be perfect for all of the people around her—her parents, friends, partner, children, co-workers, bosses, and on and on—and inside of all of that concern, her dreams were getting lost.

"I have failed myself and keep failing others, no matter how hard I try," she lamented to me one day. "It's never enough."

She had just quit a successful corporate career to start her own business. The stakes had become ten times higher, and the rollercoaster had started going much faster. Sometimes the new stressors would send her into periods where she remained cocooned on her couch, wrapped in a blanket, hiding out.

We worked first on her pattern of fear. Like many people I work with, Liana was under the mistaken impression that life should be smooth if one is taking all the right actions. As I see it, this is yet another myth of our times. Life is never easy; the trick is to learn to surf the waves. Armed with this new understanding, Liana began her 4 Step journey.

A few months later, she launched a tech start-up that builds software to understand human emotions. She became a businesswoman in what she perceived as being a "man's world," and she needed even more resilience and tenacity to succeed. Still, the old Liana—the one that would have crumbled under this weight—was gone.

She started writing and speaking about empathy and how businesses need to "grow heart" to succeed. She hired staff across three continents and took on the role of CEO in her swiftly-growing company. She started negotiating tough contracts with high-powered executives, doing television and radio interviews, firing partners who didn't quite measure up and doing all of it with the cool confidence available from knowing how to create optimal patterns. In her first year, she became the first female winner of an International Start-Up Competition and stepped out onto a stage in Amsterdam to receive her award. In her second year in business, her company was one of five female-owned companies to be awarded venture capital. Today she continues to spread her message about the need to build another kind of business - one based on collaboration, integrity and higher purpose.

The success of these two women had nothing to do with their starting points. As both of their stories demonstrate, they didn't set out to accomplish the level of achievement they eventually acquired. Even more to the point, both of them, at the start of their journeys, never would have dreamed that they were capable of what they are now accomplishing.

Liana and Aubrey's case studies illustrate something else that is truly remarkable about the human identity: The "I" does not have to be a singular "I"; it can, by way of the 4 Steps, expand to the level of the group. Let's explore this together in the next chapter.

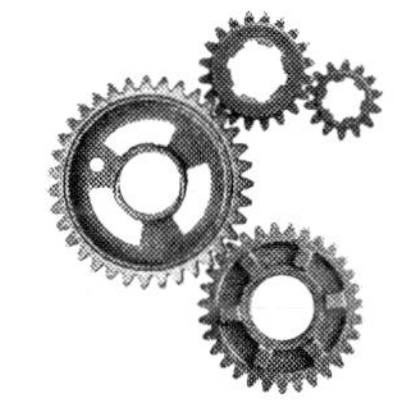

Chapter 14: The Ever-Expanding "I"

Most popular self-development programs place a great deal of emphasis on polishing and perfecting the self. We strive to become extraordinary; for example, we vision board in efforts to distinguish personal goals, we work on becoming leaders or "team players," and we look to enhance our strengths and downplay our weaknesses.

The 4-Step Repatterning Technique approach is different. As you use it daily, over time, you will notice your "I" softens and your overall emphasis on your "I" diminishes.

I noticed this a couple of years into using the 4 Steps. Whereas at one time, I would have gotten defensive or felt the need to justify my actions, I then felt only curiosity when someone got upset with me or questioned me. Whereas prior I would have felt pride at people's acknowledgements of me, I then felt only pleased that I was able to help.

Sometimes it is interesting watching the reactions of people around me now. Some of us cannot comprehend a world in which the "I" softens, and the goal of the group takes priority over personal reward. People are all-too-often suspicious.

I once said to a group of workshop participants, who I had just invited on a full-year journey of transformation, "Are you aware that I don't care if you sign up or not?" I did not say it defensively, or with malice. My individual self didn't care because its sole focus was on what was best for the group. If the other person would benefit from what I was offering, then my "I" was delighted to share its gifts; if the other wouldn't benefit, then my "I" desired what was best for that person. There was no personal agenda present.

This expansion of self is what some people in the past have come across by happenstance, or perhaps through prayer or meditation. Although I in no way mean to compare myself to the historical greats, it is the Gandhis, the Martin Luther Kings and the Mother Theresas of this world who have, through deep contemplation and self-reflection, come to an expanded sense of self that includes others.

The Dalai Lama once appealed to the scientific community: Could they research a methodology that would speed up the effects of meditation? He asked this because he was aware that meditation decreases the typical emphasis on self-centred interests and increases our level of compassion, both for others and for the planet.

Interestingly, despite decades of meditating, I never reached the diminished emphasis on self-interest on which the Dalai Lama had based his appeal. My emphasis remained on me and "mine." But with only a few years of consistent application of the 4-Step Repatterning Technique, I came to understand what the great masters of the past were trying to impart on us.

Patterns pulled from the past bring an experience of separation, and separation brings problems. These problems have become so commonplace that we think of them as innate to our humanity, but I have come to realise that none of this conflicted experience is necessary. The problems are: fear, self-doubt, anxiety, body image issues and concerns about one's looks, shame, the desire to hide our flaws, the need to lie or cover up our mistakes, defensiveness, greed, perfectionism, the need to justify, irritation with another person's shortcomings, superiority, and so on.

The 4-Step Repatterning Technique eliminates all of this, but not in the way that you might assume. It is not that you become the opposite of these problems—as in becoming extraordinary, special, outstanding, generous, and such—because all of that is still based in you being separate from others. Rather, it is in the softening of your "I" that results from the technique: Your identity expands to include not just yourself, but also the group around you.

To understand how and why this works, we need to return to the sequence of a pattern. Recall that it looks like this:

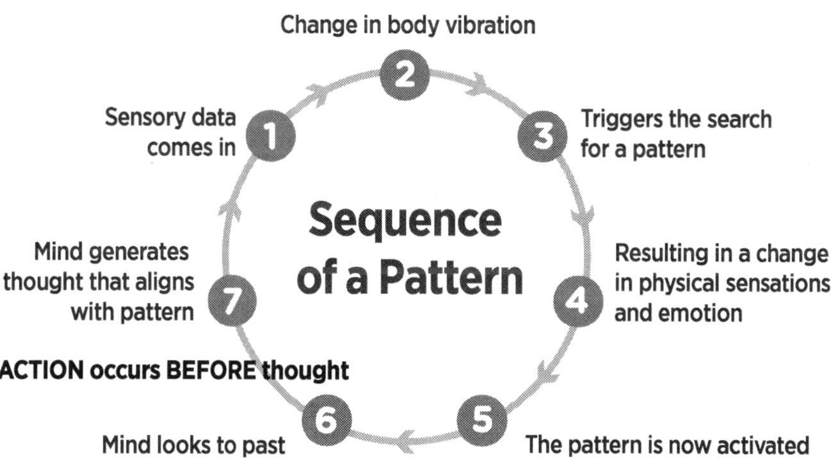

That is, this is the sequence of events that occurs when your pattern box is full, and you are pulling a pattern from your past to deal with your current situation. But what happens when there is no pattern in the box? In other words, what is the effect of a deconstructed pattern on this sequence?

When you deconstruct a pattern the effect on the sequence is as follows: Sensory data (#1) comes in through your senses, (#2) changes your body's vibration and (#3) triggers the search for a pattern. However, because you have deconstructed the old pattern, the search turns up empty (the deconstructed pattern has left a void in the pattern box). Therefore, instead of triggering the old physical sensation and emotion that you would have experienced in the past (#4), the absence of a pattern causes the need to generate a brand new physical sensation and emotion -- sensations that now align with your body vibration that is reflecting the actual situation as it is.

The process of generating a brand new pattern has now begun (#5), and your subconscious is alerted that a change is occurring and that different action is required. With no past pattern available to reference(#6), your subconscious must, in turn, look to what is happening at this moment (in this situation) to determine the needed action.

The action then takes place, and thought is generated that explicates that action (#7). The new sequence, therefore, looks like the following diagram.

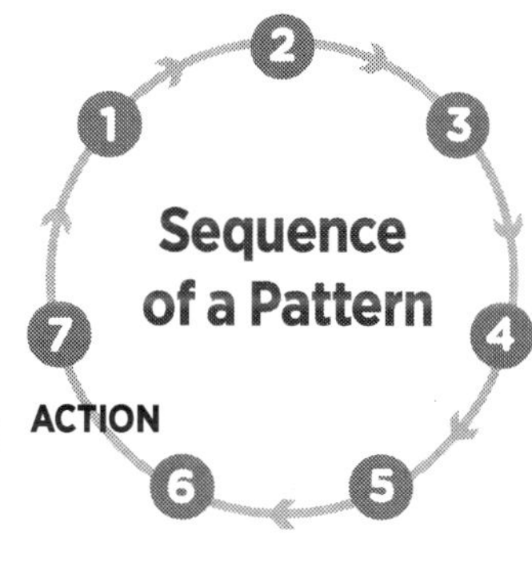

1. Sensory Data
2. Changes in Body Vibration
3. The search for a pattern turns up none, triggers the need for a new pattern
4. Instead of turning to the box, the pattern generates a physical sensation/emotion based on the actual body vibration occurring now
5. The process of generating a brand new pattern begins.
6. The subconscious looks first to the past, but with no past pattern available, it now turns its attention to the present situation in efforts to make sense out of the body's reaction

ACTION occurs before THOUGHT

7. The mind generates a thought that aligns with what is going on at this moment.

Now we get to the exciting part. What your about to read may sound strange at first. Please be patient as you learn a whole new and delightful way of understanding yourself.

Keeping in mind that every one of your patterns arises as an identity, and that a pattern has three parts (physical sensation, emotion and thought), where is your identity between the time the search for a pattern turned up blank (at #3) (i.e. the moment that the old pattern was dropped), and the completion of the new pattern with the generation of a new thought (at #7)?

The answer is surprising because your "I" (your identity) is suspended until the completion of the pattern which only takes place at #7. Your thought, (the one that solidifies your identity at #7) the one that is not available to you until the full sequence is complete, will then be a reflection of the newly-created action that you just took.

And herein lies the gold, because that new pattern (the newly formed intertwining of physical sensation and thought, which brings with it a new experience of you) generates a "you" that extends beyond the self-considerations of your old box of patterns.

Here is the full benefit of the 4-Step Repatterning Technique: The action that the new pattern took, came before you consciously became aware that you took that action. And because it is now a brand new pattern, it is aligned not only with you and your needs but also with the group and the group's needs. All newly generated patterns take care of you and those around you, at the same time.

To understand how this happens, let's revisit what comprises the present moment (i.e. what exists in the body vibration (#2)). Recall in *Step Four—Trust*, we discussed the answer to the question, "What is in the here and now?" Recall that the moment consists of the following three things:

1. **The vast warehouse which houses all of your past experiences.**
2. **The goal that you are trying to achieve.**
3. **Other people who will be affected by the action your pattern is taking/will take**

Now let's consider this. Your right hemisphere does not prioritise any one of these three items over the other (refer back to Chapter 12 to review the difference between the hemispheres). On this side of the brain, you are not separate from everyone else, your needs are no more or no less important; you are instead, part and parcel of the whole, a whole that equally includes you and those around you.

The left hemisphere (the place where your existing pattern box is stored) is only able to take you and your needs into account. Recall that the left hemisphere re-presences the past. It overrides what is here at this moment, with what it perceives to be here based on its past experiences. A past-created pattern can only be about you because it was created for a different time and situation in which the only common denominator between now and then, is you. And so as you remove this pattern, and cause your subconscious to tap into the right hemisphere to generate an action for this situation, you access the way of perceiving that your right hemisphere provides.

Tap into the right, and you automatically, innately, naturally take care of your own interests and those of the group, equally, simultaneously, just simply because this is the nature of your brain, not because of anything that you need do to cause it. It happens because (as the right hemisphere knows) you have never been separated from anyone else, (not really), you have always been patterns and patterns can be pulled from the past, or generated in the present. Either way, action still comes before conscious awareness. Either way, you take action, before you become consciously aware that you are taking that action. And then, your mind does what your mind does: It generates a thought that justifies the action already taken. Since the action includes the whole, the "you" that gets birthed arises naturally as one who is able to take the best action to support the group.

THE BENEFITS OF GROUP CONSCIOUSNESS

When I first met Rose, she had just stepped into a management role at a non-profit organisation. One of her numerous responsibilities was to oversee the staff meetings.

It didn't take too many meetings before Rose realised that she was losing control of the meetings. After a bit of sleuthing, she recognised that she was allowing the men in the room to dominate the agenda. Feeling disempowered around the high profile men, she was allowing the meetings to go in the direction they wanted them to go in instead of in the direction she needed them to go in.

Rose became familiar enough with Repatterning to know that the best viable solution was to deconstruct her patterns rather than to blame either herself or the men in the room. She deconstructed right up to the start of the next meeting.

Afterwards, Rose was pleased with how well the meeting had gone. She was also pleasantly surprised by the differences she saw in Jake, one of the men in the organisation. Jake, who was in charge of major gifts, was often rather aggressive. Before deconstructing, Rose would have said that he was outwardly hostile toward her, rolling his eyes, sitting stone-faced in the meetings, or deliberately undermining what she would say. Rose sounded hesitant when she told me about her most recent meeting: "Do you know," she confided, "he was almost pleasant."

Perhaps, had we been flies on the wall, we might have been able to pinpoint what was causing the different dynamics that day. Was Rose standing a little straighter? Was her tone a little less hesitant? Were her directions clearer? We will never know because, frankly, Rose doesn't know, and neither for that matter, does anyone else who was sitting at that table. Rose was left only with the understanding that the meeting was different, and the rest of the group was likely unaware of anything being different at all.

What makes Repatterning so unique and so effective is that Rose's actions now served the group as a whole. Her new pattern took into account the totality of the dynamics and responded effectively to ensure that she met everyone's needs.

This altered Rose: Her pattern (her new identity) now responds intuitively, knowing what to do and what to say to direct meetings effectively. Rose couldn't have done this consciously. Consciously trying to make things right is a messy way of leading. It requires that we chastise or cajole others, that we seek out ways to compromise and communicate, that we make things wrong, and that we make things right. None of this is effective because all of this assumes that what the old pattern is informing us about the situation is somehow correct, even though it is bringing us a partial picture of the whole.

However, Rose is not without resources. The moment itself contains the answers she needs because the answers are birthed out of her vast warehouse of past experiences, combined with the goal of the meeting and the needs of the group. Rose, therefore, has only to create the opening for the optimal pattern to arise by way of letting go of her past-created patterns.

Then, a pattern gets created in the present and brings with it a unique experience. The focus is not on you, or self, at all (although the self is equally taken care of by the new pattern). As the awareness of self softens, so does your experience of "me" and "them." Your identity is suspended, waiting for your thoughts that will inform you as to who you are. It is not that your "I" disappears; rather, your "I" is just one more part of the whole, equally important and equally relevant to everyone and everything else.

There is remarkable freedom in this, along with remarkable compassion, ability to speak openly, curiosity born out of a desire to truly understand the other person's perspective, listening, presence, peace of mind and joy, all of which come naturally and without to need for 'you' to do anything but deconstruct.

As you let go of your past-created patterns, you let go of all attachment to the illusion of "you," or self, as separate from others.

The Buddha attempted to tell us over 2,500 years ago, we human beings are "no self." Few people have grasped the significance of this teaching. "No self " is not selflessness; it is not emptiness nor sacrifice. "No self " provides the means to arise anew into a situation instead of arriving there from the past. It provides the totality of the situation and therefore, the optimal response. Best of all, it is an experience of letting go of individual concerns, where the separation of self and other dissolves, and the "I" ceases to be the centre of its own universe.

THE BENEFITS OF SURRENDER

I had turned on the radio at the tail end of a Quirks and Quarks episode. *Quirks and Quarks* [4] is the radio science program of the Canadian Broadcasting Corporation. This award-winning show presents the latest discoveries in the natural sciences. I tuned in to Bob McDonald interviewing Dr Andrew Newberg, and the topic of inquiry was what happens in our brains when we surrender. I sat up and took notice.

Dr Newberg said:

> *When we look at the brains of [the] individuals who feel [the] feeling of surrender, there's an area of [the] brain right behind our forehead (our frontal lobe) that actually starts to shut down. And this is very interesting because the frontal lobe normally turns on when we are purposefully, willfully doing something, when we are concentrating on something, or when we are trying to make a connection with something. But in practices [in which surrender is present]...instead of seeing an increase in frontal lobe activity, we actually see a drop of the activity or a decrease of activity in that area.*

McDonald interrupted to inquire if any other part of the brain was affected when one surrendered.

Dr Newberg answered with:

> *We have another area of our brain called the parietal lobe, located at the back of our brain, and this normally takes our sensory information and helps to establish our sense of self. What we propose and, have found a substantial amount of evidence for, is that when a person loses their sense of self, they actually feel that the boundary between themselves and the rest of the world starts to dissipate. Then the loss of the sense of self is concomitantly associated with a decrease of activity in this area.*

McDonald: *When you say it's "rewiring" our brain, what's the brain doing there?*

Dr Newberg answered:

> *It's almost as if we have a big filing cabinet, and our frontal lobes help to keep that filing cabinet in order so that all of our ideas about jobs and relationships, etc....are all set in a certain way. And when that frontal lobe activity drops, suddenly all the controls are taken off, and all of the different ways in which we think about things get thrown up into the air. Then when they come down, we ultimately have a whole different set of beliefs. This is actually seen in the neuro-wiring of our brain: the neurons in our brain can connect and reconnect with each other, they can connect thousands of different ways with other neurons, and we can ultimately affect and change the ways in which we perceive our world [and] perceive our reality.*

Here was scientific proof that *Step Three—Surrender* is essential if we are going to step out of one identity and into another. Surrender, positioned within the 4-Step technique, becomes a vital part of the whole and is what enables us to transcend this "I." As Dr Newberg explains it, surrendering has the effect of tossing all of our individual beliefs up into the air and rearranging them so that they become a whole different set of beliefs.

Step Three is challenging for many, precisely because it has to be. It is about doing the deep work needed to transcend our individual selves and (automatically) coming to a new understanding that includes the group. As I mentioned earlier, the consistent application of the technique has the effect of expanding each one of us from individual consciousness to group consciousness. Group consciousness is the ability to take care of the whole. It takes into account all of the members of the group and what is best for all, instead of what is best for one or the other.

How do we typically form groups? Don't we tend to come together over a mutually agreed-upon goal or objective? Following that, are we not expected to commit to that goal and then make compromises or even personal sacrifices in efforts to advance the group in the direction of that goal?

As you cross the threshold from individual consciousness to group consciousness, just how ineffective and unnecessary this approach is, becomes visible. The actions that flow out of a deconstructed pattern *automatically align with the best interests of the group* (a group that now includes you). Inside a group in which all members are deconstructing, your needs and your wants are automatically taken care of at the level of the group.

There is a group of us who work together to support the sharing of the 4-Step Repatterning Technique. At one point, we were struggling to find the time to work on our own businesses (we are all entrepreneurs) and support the participants of the 4-Step programs at the same time.

Here is what a traditional approach to such a problem would likely look like: We would start with the objective of supporting the participants. Then we would come together to brainstorm how to do that in the limited amount of time allotted to the problem. We would make sacrifices: "You skip this part of your business, and I'll do this instead," or would ask the participants to make sacrifices: "We'll cut down the number of calls to every other week – they'll understand."

Being Pattern Makers, we did none of that.

We each started with our individual concerns, and then we supported each other in deconstructing these concerns.

What resulted was the birth of a new program that equally took care of the business, took into consideration the needs of the participants, included times for the group members to work on their own businesses, and provided additional income for all involved.

The solution was not like anything we would have considered in a brainstorming session. The solution was seamless. Not a single compromise was being asked of anyone.

So how do you create group consciousness? Paradoxically is the answer. Start by addressing each member's concerns. Look at each person's desires, fears, self-doubts, money issues, time issues, and so on. Address all of those using the 4-Step Repatterning Technique until there comes a time when a fundamental state change takes place, and the subconscious crosses the divide from the individual to the group.

Let the technique work its magic. Let your personal concerns be the indication that it is time to deconstruct, and you won't have to work to reach the stage of group consciousness – it will happen organically.

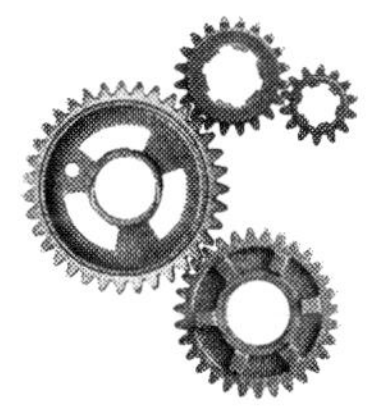

Chapter 15: Relationships Under Repair

I have given you an in-depth look at how the 4-Step Repatterning Technique compares to recent research in neuroscience and the kind of results that are available when using the technique, including the shift from individual to group consciousness. Now I'd like to share with you how the technique can shift your relationships. I'll start by sharing two stories.

THE VICTIM

Tom was bullied as a child by his older brother. His brother, being six years older, was of course much bigger and stronger. As a child, Tom would find himself all-too-often under the enormous bulk of his brother as he sat on top of him, laughing at Tom's helpless attempts to escape. Tom grew up hating his brother.

As with many family patterns, the story didn't end there. Tom had a son, and as he grew up, Tom often found himself at odds with his little boy. As is typical of many eight-year-olds, his son often wanted to horse around with his father, sometimes in ways that made Tom feel very angry.

Of course, he tried all the usual parenting tricks: time outs, firm communication, and walking away when he could; however, nothing worked. The boy persevered, and Tom continued to feel helpless anger.

When I met Tom, he hadn't been in touch with his brother for over a decade.

As Tom deconstructed his pattern toward his son, he saw the connection between the situation with his son and that of the past involving his brother. He switched his focus to deconstructing the pattern he held for his brother.

What happened next came as a surprise.

Tom realised that his brother had only wanted to play with him. Forgiveness followed.

THE BULLY

When I met Sharon, she would often recount times when her twin sister had been openly aggressive toward her. Initially, Sharon believed that her sister was to blame for this conflict. Sharon herself was very close to their mother, and her sister was often absent, leaving Sharon to provide the sole care for their mother as she aged. Sharon blamed her sister bitterly for this, accusing her of being selfish for not wanting to contribute.

It was not easy for Sharon to even begin to apply the 4-Step Repatterning Technique on the patterns she held for her sister because of how strongly she felt towards her. However, kudos to Sharon: She persisted. Over time, a new picture of events emerged.

As Sharon created new patterns using the technique, she came to the startling conclusion that it was she, along with her mother, who had kept her sister at bay for so many years. She became aware of the subconscious way that the two of them had colluded to have her sister be continually left out. She became aware of all the times she had not informed her sister about the family's happenings.

She came to see that her sister's aggression was simply an ineffective attempt to communicate her feelings of abandonment.

This new understanding of past events came without any feelings of self-blame either. Sharon was able to step back and perceive the big-picture without the blame and shame that typically accompanies such insight.

EMPATHY, COMPASSION AND THE 4-STEP REPATTERNING TECHNIQUE

As divorce rates skyrocket, families break down, and conflicts escalate into wars, bringing the 4-Step Repatterning Technique to relationships has never been more needed as it is today.

What always surprises and delights me about the 4-Step process is the total empathy for all parties, including (and this is often the most surprising part) ourselves.

Isn't conflict all about fault-finding? Don't we need to assign blame? Shouldn't we apologise or force an apology from the other side? Repatterning demonstrates that none of this is necessary because, so far as an optimal pattern is concerned, finding blame is pointless.

From a holistic perspective, there is never anybody to blame.

Only an optimal pattern can dance in paradox. Only an optimal pattern can take responsibility for the actions taken in the past, even if those actions hurt someone else, without assigning blame to them; likewise, only an optimal pattern can accept the hurt done to us without assigning blame to the other. The whole includes a lot more than the individual parts, and an optimal pattern can take in the whole, plus the parts. In context, there is no blame; there is only compassion.

My phone rang one day.

"I had to call you Adele," Cindy said, giggling into the phone. "The funniest thing just happened." Cindy was new to the 4-Step Repatterning Technique and had been applying the 4 Steps for just a few weeks.

She began by saying, "Twenty years ago, we moved to a new house. The kids were just babies at the time - two of them were still in diapers. The house we moved into had an ant infestation, and so there I was with three kids and ants everywhere, living out of boxes, and, in the middle of all of this, my husband tells me he has to go on a business trip.

"He came back two weeks later. I'd been dealing with everything. And when he got back, he happened to be sitting at the dining room table, and I happened to catch a glimpse of the back of his neck. And it was tanned!"

I didn't understand what that meant, but I didn't want to interrupt.

"I've been mad ever since. Well not every day of course, but every once in a while he'll say something that triggers that memory of him going off golfing while I was home with ants and boxes and diapers, and it makes me furious." I smiled. Golfing – now, I understood.

"So it happened again," she continued. "Our youngest daughter moved out this week, and he said to me, 'Isn't it nice that we are now empty nesters?' I don't know why, but just him saying that triggered that old memory and I felt that surge of anger all over again. I was so mad I burst into tears.

"But you know, I remembered what you said about the 4 Steps, so I just said to myself, *I'm just going to try that Adele thingy!*" I chuckled at that one.

"So, I did. I did exactly what you said. I went to the bathroom, and I did the 4 Steps.

"Mid sob! *Mid sob*, Adele! I stopped crying in mid sob! I was so surprised; I started looking for my anger. I actually tried to get it back. But I couldn't find it.

"So do you know what I did?" she giggled impishly. "I phoned a friend. I recounted the whole thing: the move, the ants, the business trip, the golfing -- I was trying to get angry again, but I couldn't. It's totally gone!"

Sitting in your pattern box is expensive, both for yourself and for those around you. An unworkable pattern has no access to what is beyond itself. As I've mentioned throughout the book, it can only think in terms of either/or: either you or the other person/people around you: *Either I let my guard down and the other person wins, or I keep my guard up, and I win*. Meanwhile, nobody wins, and everyone suffers.

Compassion is the ability to rise above a situation and understand all perspectives at the same time. It requires that you attempt to feel and think as you presume the other person might be thinking and feeling, something that is often referred to as, 'putting yourself in the other person's shoes'. This is a difficult thing to do when we are angry. To truly understand another, you must first rid yourself of the limited perspective derived from that past-created pattern. Remember that group consciousness does not start with the group; it starts with you.

Putting yourself first is directly opposed to the typical approach: As people form groups, they start by defining group objectives, group goals and group dynamics. And whether that is a group of two, such as in marriage, or a group of thousands, makes no difference. Members of the group are always expected to make sacrifices if their needs conflict with the group needs. Group members compromise and in that compromise resentments build up; resentments that eventually lead to arguments, divorce, broken relationships and war-torn countries.

With the 4 Steps, compromise is unnecessary and unneeded. However, why this is so can only be understood through paradox, as I mentioned earlier. There was little point in my saying to Sharon that she was the one who was ostracising her sister; her pattern could not even begin to entertain that fact. Hints in this direction were met with justifications, defensiveness and the further seeking of evidence in support of her sister being the "evil" one. To Sharon, the pattern was real; and so we started there.

As Sharon took on one pattern at a time, applying the 4 Steps to each memory and each belief about her sister, a new Sharon started to emerge. Her relationship with her sister was only one piece of the whole. Sharon came to realize that she had a pattern for "rescuing" that positioned her as the caregiver for her mother and son; a pattern for "I'm the bad one" that had her consistently trying to prove her self-worth; and a pattern for "I'm not heard," which had her always speaking and never listening. These patterns were not exclusive to her relationship with her sister, although they certainly contributed to it.

No one relationship ever stands alone; each one is an intertwining of numerous others born out of cultural patterns, family patterns, peer patterns and sibling patterns. We are interconnected, interrelated beings who are the sum of all of our various interactions with others. For Sharon, this meant that as she took on her own patterns, she began healing the patterns within her family that had likely existed for centuries. Although she was but one cog in the wheel, that one cog had an enormous influence on the whole.

Sharon's new patterns caused unforeseeable changes within her family. Her mother, who had isolated herself for years, began to socialize and sought out friends. Her brain-injured son was able to start taking better care of himself and his possessions. Her husband transformed, her friends transformed, and her relationship to money transformed.

Her family became more cohesive, each member experiencing more confidence, happiness and capability, based solely on Sharon's willingness to take on her own individual patterns. What is important to note, however, is that Sharon did not set out to heal her family; she set out to heal *herself.*

In her own words, Sharon explains it this way: "In the past I had attempted to heal the rift between my sister and me. I took a personal development program that made me feel terribly guilty. They pushed me to apologise to my sister, so I did. It was a disaster. I was trying to put a band-aid on a gaping wound.

"Now, as I look back, I see why that attempt didn't work. The patterns were generational. My father was one of a set of twins who didn't speak to each other. In my family, cousins didn't talk to each other; sisters didn't talk to each other and mothers didn't talk to their children – we were all positioned by jealousy, comparison and trying to be the favourite. The patterns don't belong to my sister and me; they're patterns that have been repeated, by generation after generation. So yes, I could have kept *trying,* but I would have kept *failing*.

"With Repatterning, I wasn't *trying* to do anything; I just took on deconstructing my patterns about my sister. I didn't do it to fix anything. I did it because I wasn't happy. But then something strange happened: I stopped justifying, and I was no longer defensive. Not just about my sister, but about anything. In the end, I realised the difference between Repatterning and other techniques is that there is nothing to remember and nothing to apply. I am just different now."

To create new patterns, and impact the world around us, we must start with our own, dare I say, selfish, self-centred, self-absorbed views of the world. We must start at the only place we *can* start: with the views of ourselves provided by our past-created-patterns that brings with it the experience of being separate, isolated, misunderstood, conflicted, victimised, bullied, wronged, and the like. We begin here, not only because this is the most effective place to begin, but because there is nowhere else to begin.

Messages that inform us "something is wrong," interpreted correctly, beckon to us and invite us to look within. Our suffering motivates us to want to end that suffering, but as we put an end to our suffering, we support those around us to do the same.

So go ahead. Give yourself permission to be self-centred, to be angry, or to be hurt, and then apply the 4 Steps in that direction. After all, it is only a pattern.

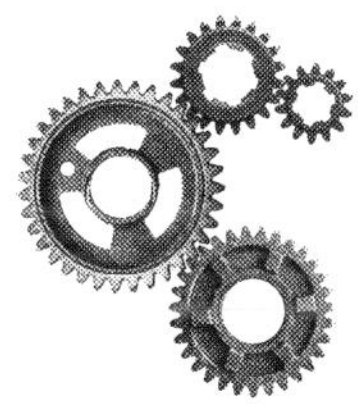

Chapter 16: Trailblazers in a New Land

Imagine that you are alone in a small boat. The gentle rocking of the waves causes you to fall asleep, and you drift lazily through your dreams.

Suddenly you wake up to find that the boat has been adrift for a long time. You are in the middle of the ocean, and there is no land in sight. There are no other boats, no birds to indicate where the shore is and nothing that will allow you to navigate. How do you feel? Excited? Scared? Panicked?

André Gide once said, "Man cannot discover new oceans unless he has the courage to lose sight of the shore."

We have just lost sight of the shore.

I suggested earlier that it won't be long before it is widely accepted that to take a new action, you will need to change your patterns. As I write this book, however, this understanding is only just coming to light.

Up until now, techniques such as the 4 Step Repatterning Technique have not been necessary. Throughout much of history, progress was steady. Life did not require new patterns. The patterns created in childhood were enough to carry you through your entire life. In a world in which change is slow, it is easy to adapt by using existing patterns.

Those days are now gone.

Today, the world has sped up, and change is only getting faster. To navigate through these changing times you will have to change -- no, not just change, that is an oversimplification -- you will need to transform – you will need to change not just once in a while, but continuously, over and over again.

That will require two things: 1. the ability to embrace the unknown, and 2. a loss of the concept of 'self.'

As the Buddha determined 2500 years ago, the definition of self has always been limiting. Human beings were never supposed to be fixed beings. You have never been what you are educated to believe yourself to be: one singular, individual identity, separate and distinct from seven billion other separate and individual identities. You have always been patterns, and a pattern can either be separate, or it can be group depending on whether it was created in the past, or created now.

In large part, this technique is arising now because our understanding of 'identity' is no longer being supported by the current global experience.

A new world view is emerging, and it rides in on the back of global communication channels made possible by the internet, global issues such as global warming and mass extinction, global fears such as terrorism, and new theories made possible by changes in neuroscience and philosophy.

Although it is not widely recognised, we are already positioned in the unknown, looking out on a brand new world. This new world pulls for collaboration and invites every individual to put aside individual concerns in favour of a holistic perspective.

But how do we do that inside an existing box of patterns that only has access to 'me' and 'mine'...inside a box of existing patterns created in your past, bringing you a singular perspective that is innately self-centred?

The answer is: We cannot.

And so, in the face of a radically new world, a radically new philosophy is emerging. This new philosophy will no longer position the individual at the centre of his or her own existence. It will elevate the individual to the level of the group. Every action taken by the individual will then equally support you, the group and the planet.

Before we can do that, we must get comfortable in the unknown. This moment—this now—can never be known; it is always arising into this present moment – it never arrives there from the past.

The only way to navigate the unknown is to become it. We, too, must arise and stop arriving.

Walk through any door, not knowing who you are to be, what actions are required, how you are to behave, or what you are to believe. Walk through every door as a vehicle; as an opening into which the optimal pattern can, and will, arise.

As you master this, you will flow, as effortlessly as the moment itself flows, and as unknowable as this present moment is.

So use this technique. Use it for as long as you need to use it. Use it to carry you through these changing times until you get to the other side.

Please don't underestimate the journey you are about to embark on. The current emphasis on the self is pervasive, and the unknown looms large. In the beginning, few will get it. Those who do will be liberated.

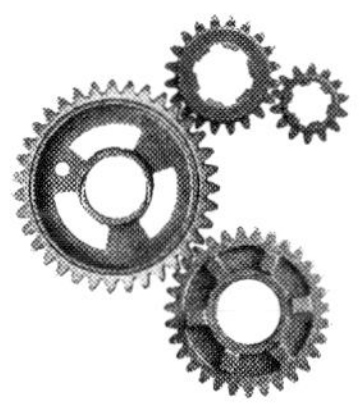

Appendix: Repatterning Tips

TIP # 1: Start with a list.

Eventually, as you become better at Repatterning, you will be able to apply the 4 Steps when you are in the middle of a conflicted situation. However, to get to that stage takes mastery of the 4-Step Repatterning Technique. To begin, therefore, make a list of your actions, behaviours and beliefs as they relate to one area of your life that isn't working.

Then, twice a day, refer to the list and deconstruct a pattern that is under one of the line items. Take it one pattern at a time, and soon you will notice things changing in that area.

TIP # 2: On the mat versus off the mat.

If you are using the 4 Steps while in conflict, you are applying a more advanced use of the technique. It is easier, therefore, to start with the list (as explained in tip #1). Working from a list is what I call "working off the mat." On and off the mat is a wrestling metaphor. Wrestlers, wrestle on the mat. The mat is where the real match takes place. Practice (off the mat) happens before the match takes place. You are "on the mat" when you are caught up in the situation, and the action that the pattern takes is already in play. "Off the mat" occurs when you use a list to consider the situation. When you work from a list you don't wait until you are in an argument with your mother (for example) to begin to apply the 4 Steps. Instead, you think about the last time you had an argument with her and then get in touch with the pattern that is running now, as it relates to that argument.

TIP #3: Be consistent.

Deconstruct patterns twice a day, every day. Consistent application of the 4 Steps is required to get lasting results and to change deeply ingrained patterns.

TIP #4: Integrate this technique into your life.

Ideally, you want to integrate Repatterning into your life. In the beginning, you might want to start with an observation journal; however, don't become reliant on it. As soon as you can, let go of the need to record your patterns. After that, try Repatterning when you are walking, driving a car, on the bus, or doing routine household chores. The more you can make Repatterning a part of your daily life, the better your results will be, and you will then be able to move to the next stage of Repatterning, which is to do it while doing complex tasks.

TIP #5: Do not deconstruct the same pattern more than three times in a row.

When applying the 4 Steps, you come to the question of shift, no-shift or trap. You will be returning to the place of surrender if you encounter no-shift or trap. Don't go through this loop more than three times. To do so would be to strive for a shift and therefore, you will no longer be in the space of surrender. Just let it go for the moment and return to it the next time you go to deconstruct.

TIP #6: Enjoy the plateaus, but don't rest too long.

As you consistently apply the 4 Steps, you will find that there are times where everything in your life starts working, and it all feels effortless. It is tempting at this time to stop using the technique. The important thing is not to get complacent.

These plateaus, as I like to call them, indicate that all the new patterns you have just created are now workable. If you should stop deconstructing, however, this new box of patterns will also become obsolete. Situations are always evolving, and your patterns need to evolve with them. So enjoy the plateaus, but don't rest there too long. Set a new goal, and keep challenging yourself to take on bigger and bigger goals so you can keep expanding into group consciousness and eventually universal consciousness.

TIP #7: The proof is always in your results.

Regardless of what happens as you apply the 4 Steps, the evidence that you are doing it correctly is always in your results. Don't mistakenly think that just because you are consistently getting shifts, that you are doing it right because this will have you striving to get a shift. Likewise, don't mistakenly think that if you are not getting a shift, that you are doing it wrong. Shift or no-shift is no indication of success.

The only determination that you are on the right track is the results that you are getting in your life.

TIP #8: Put aside all other methodologies for the time being.

To get the full benefits of this technique, you will need to put aside all other techniques and methodologies. Repatterning does not integrate well with other techniques. Most methodologies require you to determine beforehand the results you desire, whereas Repatterning requires you to step into the unknown. Because patterns always gravitate toward the known, other methods will always override this one. Therefore, if you're going to give this one a try, you will need to put aside anything else for the time being.

TIP #9: Expect to drift off in the beginning.

During the space of surrender in Step Three, you may find yourself drifting off from time to time. You can expect to drift in the beginning. Please be patient with yourself. It will stop so long as you don't make it wrong and just keep gently bringing yourself back to the task at hand.

TIP #10: Don't be intimidated by overwhelm.

In the beginning, you may experience overwhelm. The patterns might feel too large or as if there are too many. This is normal. Keep in mind that no matter how big a pattern feels, it is still just a pattern (an intertwined physical sensation, emotion and thought). Likewise, remember that no matter how numerous your patterns feel, it is still just one pattern at a time. As you start applying the technique more and more, overwhelms naturally dissipate and, in time, disappear altogether.

TIP #11: Expect resistance and do it anyway.

Your existing patterns do not want anything to do with these 4 Steps. Somewhere deep in your psyche, your pattern box knows that this technique is powerful. It will, therefore, resist doing this technique in efforts to keep you safe (remember the thing that your patterns resist the most is the unknown). Therefore, expect resistance to come up as part and parcel of this technique and then apply the 4 Steps anyway.

And just as a by-the-way, after nine years of doing this technique, my patterns still resist. I see it as a good sign that the technique works.

TIP #12: Don't look for insights.

Insights are cheap. Although fresh ways of thinking can sometimes support you on your journey, insights rarely lead to lasting change. Try to catch the need to analyse or understand the trap, and instead go straight to applying the 4 Steps. That is where the gold is.

NEXT STEPS

For additional support in applying the 4 Step Repatterning Technique, the SHIFT-Kit is available at www.AdeleSpraggon.com/SHIFTKit. The SHIFT-Kit includes the following: SHIFT: The Companion Guide, a workbook of daily, bite-size activities divided over the six-week journey; Pattern Identification Cards so you can easily identify your patterns; The 4 Steps on a fold-out wallet card for easy reference; Guided Audio Instructions for deconstructing on the go, SHIFT email support for daily motivation and inspiration, and more.

To order yours, visit www.AdeleSpraggon.com/SHIFTKit

END NOTES

Page 26: Jakes, TD. *Commitment - Full Version* https://www.youtube.com/watch?v=EJgfMYqHvT4

Page 115: Doidge, Norman. *The Brain's Way of Healing: Remarkable Discoveries and Recoveries From the Frontiers of Neuroplasticity*. New York, New York: Viking, 2015.

Page 123: McGilchrist, Iain. *The Master and His Emissary: The Divided Brain and the Making of the Western World*. New Haven: Yale University Press. 2009.

Page 155: https://www.cbc.ca/radio/quirks/sealing-chernobyl-neurotheology-gene-edited-vaccines-1.3874106/how-religious-fervour-changes-your-brain-1.3874154